DESIGNS
ON
LIFE

DESIGNS
ON
LIFE

EXPLORING THE
NEW FRONTIERS OF
HUMAN FERTILITY

by

Robert Lee Hotz

POCKET BOOKS

New York   London   Toronto   Sydney   Tokyo   Singapore

POCKET BOOKS, a division of Simon & Schuster Inc.
1230 Avenue of the Americas, New York, NY 10020

Hotz, Robert Lee.
    Designs on life: exploring the new frontiers of human fertility / by Robert
Lee Hotz.
        p.   cm.
    ISBN: 0-671-69325-5 : $21.00
    1. Fertilization in vitro, Human.   I. Title.
RG135.H67   1991
618.1'78059—dc20   91-15969
                                                                            CIP

First Pocket Books hardcover printing November 1991

10   9   8   7   6   5   4   3   2   1

FOR JENNIFER

Acknowledgments
and Sources

The core of this book is the product of in-depth interviews with more than 300 patients and practitioners at a dozen infertility clinics in the United States, England, and Australia during 1989 and 1990. Over the course of two years, I found clinicians, embryologists, and patients, some of whom endured my questions and my curiosity for weeks at a stretch, unfailingly candid and generous with their insights. Some of the techniques described in the text may be obsolete by the time this manuscript is published, so quickly does the field evolve. By examining them, however, I seek to address something more enduring: the relationship between technology and conception.

I am indebted to Jacques Cohen, who first showed me a human embryo under the microscope. In that glimpse of a few suspended cells, I saw an infinitesimal imprint of creation that, as it has for so many others, altered my life. Without his honesty and good humor, this project would not have been possible. He offered expertise, patience, and what amounted to a two-year postgraduate course in clinical embryology. I have tried to honor that debt by being, as he urged, as unsparing as possible in this consideration of the new means men and women have invented to produce their offspring.

The generosity and patience of the staff of Reproductive Biology Associates in Atlanta are beyond calculation. For two years, Dr. Joe Massey, Dr. Hilton Kort, and Dr. Carlene Elsner allowed a reporter the freedom of their clinic, to share in their successes and their failures in a demonstration of openness all the more remarkable in a field where secrecy is the norm. I thank them and their staff, including their current team of embryologists: Michael Tucker, Graham Wright, and Sharon Wiker. The clinic's success rates with embryo transfers and pregnancies is as reported to the Society for Assisted Reproductive Technology.

To the degree that this book concerns a scientific discipline, it is about the practice of human embryology. For their help in understanding their specialty, I thank Mina Alikani, Henry Malter, and Beth Talansky at the Cornell Center for Reproductive Medicine and Infertility in New York; Lucinda Veeck at the Jones Institute of Reproductive Medicine in Norfolk, Virginia; Benjamin Brackett at the University of Georgia; Alan Handyside and Karen Dawson at Hammersmith and Royal Masonic Hospitals, London; Prof. Robert G. Edwards and Michael Macnamee at Bourn Hall; Peter Braude of Cambridge University; Dr. Carla Mills and Sue Avery of the Hallam Medical Centre, London; Ian Pike at Royal Women's Hospital in Sydney, Australia; and Alan Trounson and the research staff of the Centre for Early Human Development at Monash University, Melbourne, Australia. They all generously provided me access to their laboratories and to their published and unpublished work.

When I began my research I thought, somewhat naïvely, that this was a story about technology and the scientists who managed it and that the patients who volunteered for the embryo experiments were passive participants whose role in research was controlled by the doctors and embryologists who treated them. What I discovered was that these patients are the driving force. In the end, it is in their name that this revolution in human biology has been made. And it is in large measure their energy and determination that have made it. In these couples I found depths of courage, intelligence, and wisdom. Those dozens of men and women who allowed me to intrude in their most private lives did so in the belief that their experience might prove of value to the couples who would come after them—to help them anticipate the trials of laboratory conception and to let them know that "from terrible pain, great joy can come." Many have chosen to be named in this manuscript; many more have not. Throughout the text, I have indicated the use of pseudonyms with an asterisk. All of the men and women mentioned in the text, however, are real. From them I learned that all children are experiments. I acknowledge my debt to them all.

For their willingness to open their operating rooms and staff meetings to me, I would in particular like to thank Dr. Sev Rosenwaks and his colleagues at the Cornell Center for Reproductive Medicine and Infertility; Dr. Carl Wood and his colleagues at the Epworth IVF Infertility Centre in Melbourne, Australia; Dr. Suheil Muasher, Dr. Annibal Acosta, Dr. Howard W. Jones, Jr., and Dr. Georgeanna S. Jones at the Jones Institute; Yuri Verlinsky and his colleagues at IVF Illinois

ACKNOWLEDGMENTS AND SOURCES

and the Reproductive Genetics Institute in Chicago; and Vicki Baldwin and the staff of IVF Australia at Port Chester, New York.

For their help in unraveling the laws governing the international conduct of laboratory conception, I am especially grateful to Lori Andrews of the American Bar Foundation; Veronica English of the United Kingdom's Interim Licensing Authority; D. Ann Murphy, now staff director of the government operations subcommittee of the House Committee on Energy and Commerce; the staff of the U.S. Office of Technology Assessment; and Prof. Louis Waller, Sir Leo Cussen Chair of Law, Monash University, and chairman of the Standing Review and Advisory Committee on Infertility, Victoria, Australia, who was, indeed, "present at the creation."

Mary Lynn Hemphill of the Feminist Women's Health Center in Atlanta was an invaluable resource, as was Father Norman M. Ford, S.B.D., Master of Catholic Theological College in Melbourne, Australia. I also thank the organizers and participants of the Thrower Symposium on Law and Medical Genetics at Emory University, the participants in the first International Conference on Preimplantation Genetics in Chicago, the participants in Human Genome I in San Diego and in the Nature Conference on Human Gene Therapy in Boston; the Atlanta Chapter of Resolve, and the officers of the American Fertility Society and the Society of Assisted Reproductive Technology, whose annual meetings are the single most important window into a field where technology moves so much faster than any publication schedule.

This project could not have reached print without a gifted editor to shepherd it. I have been well served in that regard by Leslie Wells, senior editor at Pocket Books, from whom I have learned, after 15 years as a daily newspaper journalist, how rewarding the relationship between an editor and a writer can be. I also thank Lisa DiMona of the Sagalyn Agency in Washington, D.C., who has been everything the best literary agent should be.

For his advice and support, I am grateful to Timothy K. Smith of *The Wall Street Journal.* For their willingness to read a manuscript in progress, I thank science writer Mike King and editorial writer Marilyn Geewax, both of *The Atlanta Journal-Constitution,* and Elizabeth Arlen in London, whose advice has been especially helpful. I also thank my two research assistants, Peg Allen-Caplan and Kathy Poulson, for their hard work.

The publisher and editors—past and present—of *The Atlanta Journal* and *The Atlanta Constitution* deserve thanks for encouraging my interest in this project and granting the leave necessary to pursue it.

—Robert Lee Hotz

Contents

Preface

Beginnings

It was a small-town Mother's Day story. She was a third-grade schoolteacher turning forty; he was a mining engineer already planning for early retirement. They lived quietly off the beaten path, at the end of a country road edged each spring with a carpet of purple thistles. Their neighbors grew sod for Atlanta's sprawling suburban housing developments or worked in one of the nearby defense plants. They were devout Baptists. "Not liberal, but not hard-shell Baptist, either," she would say in the melodious singsong of her south Georgia home.

When they married in 1972, she intended to teach only two more years, then stay home to raise the four babies they planned to have. He vowed to build them a wooden cradle with his own hands, just as he had already built their home, nestled in a stand of hardwood and pine. He purchased the plans for the cradle, but the babies never came. The couple was childless. Spring after spring, the thistles bloomed and died. The plans, curled in a tight roll on a shelf, gathered dust.

"Every month I would have dreams about holding a baby. Nightmares. I would wake up and my arms would be empty," she said.

After 17 years of marriage, at an age when some of their

friends were expecting their first grandchild, they conceived a son. "She called me at work with the news. She was crying from excitement. I had tears in my eyes. She had the morning sickness and we rejoiced at that. I first saw him in the delivery room. He was dark blue, ugly looking. He started changing colors. It was amazing," he said. "I was crying, overjoyed."

The couple lived on a loop of the Bible Belt where towns-people knew their scripture almost as well as one another's business. When they read the birth announcement in the spring of 1990, they nodded in recognition. This was Elisa-beth's New Testament story: The barren wife had been re-warded for her faith with the miracle of a child. That Sunday in church, there was passing mention from the pulpit of the power of prayer and the mysterious workings of God. On its front page, the local newspaper printed a picture of the couple and their newborn in his handmade wooden cradle—an icon of an old-fashioned American nuclear family.

In truth, it was a more exotic tableau than anyone could know. Behind the public parable is a story drawn not from the Gospel of St. Luke, but from the annals of modern high technology. What the neighbors did not learn—what the cou-ple had not even told some members of their own family— was that the child had grown from an experimental embryo. In her efforts to conceive, the mother took fertility drugs for a decade—up to 61 injections a month on occasion. Then, as a volunteer in a clinical experiment, she underwent in vitro fertilization twice, and finally experimental embryo surgery, before becoming pregnant in 1989.

Like every newborn, their child owes his existence to an accident of timing and joy; an act of will and of faith. But this child's conception was also the product of a laboratory pro-cedure so unusual that only three clinics in the world had ever attempted it. The child was the result of microsurgery carried out when he consisted of no more than a few cells floating in a flat-bottomed dish. To enhance that embryo's chances of survival, a scientist named Jacques Cohen manipulated its cells at a moment when it was no larger than a grain of sand. The child in the wooden cradle was the first to survive the embryo procedure and be delivered into his parents' arms. The news of his conception—had the townspeople been able to recognize it—appeared in a medical journal four months before his birth.

And the father was mistaken. He had first seen his child long before their encounter in the delivery room. Nine months earlier, they met in a laboratory when scientists displayed the embryos they were about to transfer from an incubator into his wife. In his excitement he had forgotten. It should be no surprise that, in the squalling newborn held aloft in a hospital nursery for his inspection, he did not recognize the four cells that had become his son.

The white stork—for centuries the traditional symbol of good fortune and newborn infants—is almost extinct. For thousands of couples, reproduction is a medical procedure, an act of passion circumscribed by legal consent forms and insurance riders. The contraceptive Pill guaranteed sex without reproduction; now science allows reproduction without sex. Conception laboratories, numbering in the hundreds, are the artificial wombs in which technicians perform the tasks assigned by nature to a woman's body.

Some population experts estimate that since the dawn of time there have been 77 billion human beings on planet Earth. In the declining years of the twentieth century, about five billion of them are alive—more than at any one time in history. About 128 million new human beings are born every year. For all their diversity of language, culture, and race, they could until recently all say they shared one thing in common—the manner of their creation. No longer. By 1990, there were thousands of people whose conception took place outside the human body. And by the year 2010, such children are expected to number a million or more.

These children are part of the crowd spawned by a commercial fertility industry that in the late 1980s generated annual gross revenues of more than $2.4 billion in the United States alone. The techniques it markets to eager conception consumers are the by-products of an unprecedented scientific investigation into the chemistry and molecular biology of human reproduction. It is a science harnessed to desperation.

Eight times a day, a child is born in the United States who

was conceived outside the womb. Worldwide, perhaps 20,000 children have been born through in vitro fertilization in the dozen years since the birth in 1978 of Louise Brown, the first child to be conceived outside the human body. At least twice that many are born every year through other laboratory conception techniques such as artificial insemination. Almost as many are stored as frozen embryos in suspended animation; dozens more are conceived through donated ova or by surrogate mothers. Despite initial fears of birth defects and gross physical abnormalities, there is little to distinguish these children biologically from their playground peers, but—ethically, emotionally, spiritually—they represent a new branching of the human family tree.

This first generation of laboratory children was conceived in a decade when society was increasingly consumed—convulsed, some would say—by a systematic reappraisal of the most fundamental questions of human sexuality and family: What is a man? A woman? How do they really differ? How many mothers can a child have? Should homosexual men and women be allowed to raise children? Should anyone be allowed to control the conduct of a pregnant woman? Is a fetus more important than the woman who carries it? When does life begin? What does it mean to be human? Is biology destiny? Does an embryo have a soul? These are the koans of conception.

Never has reproductive choice encompassed such a variety of possibilities. There might not be life after death, but, in an age of sperm banks and frozen embryos, there can be posthumous procreation. Widows sue for the right to conceive with sperm collected and frozen before their husbands died. Daughters donate eggs so that their mothers can conceive. Husbands plant their seed in rented wombs. Sisters carry their sisters' children. A grandmother in Johannesburg gives birth to her own grandchildren. A divorcing husband and wife in Tennessee fight for custody of seven embryos frozen when they were 48 hours old. In Louisville, a woman obtains a court order to stop her husband from destroying the couple's six fertilized eggs. Legislators in Australia order doctors to find a mother for two frozen embryos "orphaned" when their millionaire parents died in a plane crash. In New York, a widow sues a sperm bank for confusing the semen stored by her late husband with that from a donor of a different race. On national television, a daughter vows to conceive and then abort a fetus so that its cells can be used to treat her father's Parkinson's disease. A family conceives a baby in the hope that it can become a source of bone marrow for its cancer-stricken older sister. In England, a charitable clinic arranges for the artificial insemination of a woman who has never had sexual intercourse—to produce a virgin birth.

The uneasy questions posed by the new technology of reproduction—debated in ethics seminars, courtrooms, and syndicated talk shows—arise from the answers that doctors and patients are left to find for themselves. The federal government does not fund or regulate human embryo research or research involving laboratory conception.

For infertile couples, conception is their own private struggle, but the technology designed to aid them—the array of hormone injections, surgical procedures, genetics, and cell biology techniques used to coax the union of human egg, sperm, and uterus—is a public matter. For the men and women most directly involved, the technology creates new possibilities of procreation—and new questions of risk, guilt, and responsibility. In the society around them, the technology fuels the political conflict between private reproductive choice and public policy.

The search for individual human beginnings launched biologists, theologians, judges, and legislators to seek the humanity in ever-smaller constituent parts of a human being. Infertility specialists made the human embryo the focus of their medical practice and, as a consequence, the embryo and the unique DNA that programs its development joined the human fetus as a focus in debates on public morality and ethics. For eons, the embryo had been a cluster of cells hidden in the human womb. Exposed in its laboratory petri dish, the embryo acquired a public form. It would only be a matter of time before it acquired a court-appointed attorney.

DESIGNS ON LIFE

The womb has become a construction site; sperm and eggs the bricks and mortar. Infertile couples and scientists have quietly become the architects of their own brave new world. Theirs is a step into the future of the human family, where sex and human reproduction parted company long ago.

1

The Baby Maker

Bedded on a slide clamped to a microscope's surgical stage, the patient floated into focus—four embryonic cells wrapped in a corset of granular tissue and dwarfed by a nearby air bubble. The human embryo, only hours after its conception, was still fringed with a living corona of sperm cells. Drawn from the human body's secret inner space and magnified 1,400 times on the laboratory video monitor, it was an image that more closely resembled a distant star.

The embryo was the offspring of a California screenwriter and a psychologist. Three times in five years, the couple had tried to conceive a child outside the womb. Each time, the resulting embryos had died after they were placed inside her. Even at the most proficient clinics, almost nine of every 10 embryos conceived in the laboratory died. More than 20,000 test-tube babies had been born worldwide since 1978, but the success rate, for the millions of infertile couples in the United States, was still a measure of failure. As many as half of the infertile couples who sought treatment in the 1980s never had a baby. Half of the nation's several hundred infertility clinics never had a baby, either.

Now Jacques Cohen thought he knew why, and the California couple flew 3,000 miles to Atlanta in the hope that he was right. Early on a Sunday morning in August 1989, while they finished their breakfast in their hotel, Cohen prepared for surgery. With a whisker-thin needle, he would pierce the membrane that encapsulated the embryo under the microscope. He was not a doctor. His patient was not yet a human being. He was an embryologist—one of a handful of unfunded scientists in the United States, England, and Australia who were trying to turn the human embryo into a patient.

If the morning's experiment succeeded, Cohen would quadruple the couple's chances for a child. He also might make it easier for an unhealthy embryo to survive. He could make it more likely that the embryo would split into twins or triplets. It could deform to become Siamese twins. He might even expose it to destruction by the ravaging white blood cells of its mother's immune system. To protect the embryos, Cohen suppressed her immune system with steroids. Not even Cohen completely understood why the procedure worked. "It could be that I am completely lucky," he said. "And I could be doing the right thing for the wrong reason."

Cohen and his colleagues at Reproductive Biology Associates in Atlanta and Cornell University's Center for Reproductive Medicine and Infertility in Manhattan called their embryo operation "assisted hatching." To overcome the chemical and physical barriers preventing pregnancy, Cohen and his colleagues were learning to manipulate the moment of conception. The procedure he was perfecting in his laboratory would enable scientists to operate safely on human eggs, sperm, and embryos. In the dry understatement of the technical papers they would publish that winter, Cohen and the other researchers noted that the procedure was "useful." Dr. Sev Rosenwaks, who ran the Cornell program, saw no need to temper his enthusiasm. "It is a major, major breakthrough," he said.

From a blue-plastic box on his right, Cohen lifted a minute glass scalpel, its hair-thin blade shaped by colleague Henry Malter in the heat of a microforge, then beveled to a cutting edge with a microgrinder. WE PLUCK 'EM. YOU STUCK 'EM, read the hand-lettered label on the box; WIN AN EVENING OF DINING AND DANCING WITH JACQUES COHEN. From a white container at his left, Cohen removed a hollow glass tube, its suction tip contoured to cup the cluster of embryonic cells without damage. MALTER BRAND HOLDING PIPETTES. WE HOLD YOUR EGGS OR OUR NAME ISN'T MALTER. HUMAN SIZE, read the note on the lid. In fine print: THE MALTER PIPETTE CO. IS NOT RESPONSIBLE FOR ANYTHING.

Henry Malter, dressed in loose-fitting maroon scrub trousers, a pea green short-sleeved shirt, and pale blue surgical cap, watched curiously over Cohen's shoulder. A silver peace symbol glistened in one pierced ear. The thirty-year-old Emory University biologist specialized in the micromanipulation of human cells. Together, the two had perfected the techniques that made the embryo surgery possible. By cutting a microscopic hole in the embryo, Cohen and Malter believed they could vastly improve its chances for survival in the womb. By intervening even earlier in other cases to micromanipulate the human sperm and egg, they believed they could force the union between gametes, as the human reproductive cells are called. Despite their confidence, they were hesitant to predict the fate of the embryo before them.

"It's like every time you do it, it's an experiment with that one patient," Malter said.

As Cohen tightened the instruments in place, Malter quickly switched the channel on the video monitor. The embryo disappeared and a vintage war movie—*Back to Bataan*, airing on a commercial television broadcast—flickered in its place. Actor Lloyd Nolan hunched over a machine gun in a jungle foxhole, shouting defiance at shadows charging from the fog. Before Cohen could look up, Malter changed the channel back. The embryo reappeared.

"Hey, just checking out the other stations," he said.

Cohen pressed his eyes against the binocular eyepiece of the microscope and eased the point of the glass scalpel into view. He prepared to make the incision.

Cohen, Malter, and their colleagues would repeat the operation more than 200 times in the year to come. They had already performed three clinical trials with the technique. In every case, the volunteers were couples seeking to conceive a family—who, out of hope or out of growing despair, loaned their bodies and their gametes to science. Like all medical research, the experiment began with a patient and a patient's complaint. Many patients with a terminal illness were willing to risk the side effects of experimental drugs; childless couples would risk no less to conceive. In a way unique to their situation, they risked more than death—they gambled with new life.

Each new human embryo Cohen altered would be transferred immediately into the womb of a married woman who had volunteered for the experiment. In the first phase of the experiment, more than half the women would become pregnant. Of the first seven, two would bear triplets; two would carry twins. If the couples had chosen to become human research subjects, it was a decision they made for an unborn child, as well. In making that choice, they had little enough to guide them: faith, a newspaper clipping, the word of the doctors most directly involved, a consent form. It was a gamble. They were warned; they were on their own.

William and Lisa Fagg were ambivalent lab rats, as were John and Dana Hobart*. They consented to Cohen's embryo experiment rather than concede defeat. David and Lisa Boone volunteered knowing full well that without the aid of an endocrinologist and an embryologist she could never conceive. Susan and David Parr joined in the hopes that microsurgery would help her conceive twins, so that she would not have to go through in vitro fertilization again. After four failed attempts at laboratory conception, Pamela and Larry Roberts didn't find the micromanipulation of their embryos nearly as risky as another round of fertility drugs. Others joined Cohen's experiment out of grief and frustration. "Isn't there anything you can do to make these embryos implant?" one anguished woman begged a clinic nurse.

These couples knew the territory they traveled was only sparingly charted and that the experiment, however traumatic, was no guarantee of a child. During 1989 and 1990, the couples would pass in the clinic's corridors a dozen times and never speak. They were the strangers who waited across the aisle for the nurse to call. They were never introduced, yet they shared an intimacy known to few other men and women. Their eggs, their sperm, their embryos passed through the same hands in the same dimly lit, walk-in conception chamber. If they looked deep enough into one another's eyes, they would find a reflection of their own hope and determination.

However many infertile couples went to see a doctor, only a few—less than one percent—ended up in the hands of the laboratory embryologists. They were immigrants to the brave new world, where they were tutored in the ABC's of experimental human conception: IVF, TDI, AID, IUI, TET, GIFT, ZIFT, PROST, TOAST, DIPSI, SUZI, and FREDI. All are acronyms for laboratory procedures designed to produce a pregnancy. All have a low chance of success. The most determined couples would try as many of them as they could. These couples became the medical volunteers, a kind of infertile elite. The reproduction revolution ran on their pain. In all, couples like them spent about $70 million a year trying to do what, for so many others, simply came naturally.

The thirty-three-year-old auditor dealt out the three photographs one at a time like playing cards onto the glass-topped coffee table. Each showed a cluster of embryos. Each was a souvenir of a pregnancy that failed; each photograph was a marker for $8,000 in medical bills. They were the closest thing Susan and David Parr had to baby pictures.

The Parrs were weekend sailors who were landlocked by the effort to have a baby. To conceive, the couple tried artificial insemination seven times. Twice, Susan underwent the full regimen of hormone injections, ultrasound egg retrieval, and embryo transfer for in vitro fertilization (IVF). Twice the couple froze embryos for future use. Three times they volunteered for experimental embryo procedures. Nothing worked. "I am dependent on the technology, and that is very scary," Susan said. "If it were not for that, I would be a barren woman. In an earlier time, King Henry would have divorced me. I'd have my head cut off. Everything I am doing is experimental. I have to trust in a doctor. The one thing my husband can give me now is emotional support—that and good sperm."

On the bookshelf in the living room, between the infertility texts and videotape cassettes of her pelvic surgeries, was a paperback romance novel, its binding crimped by bite marks. She clenched the book between her teeth to stifle her groans when her husband gave her the daily hormone injections.

"It starts out with taking just one hormone pill to get pregnant. Then suddenly you are doing all these other things. I'll do whatever I have to in order to have a biological child. I'm willing to sacrifice my body. Somewhere along the line I came up with the courage," Susan said.

She rearranged the embryo photographs into chronological order. May 19, 1989. July 8, 1989. October 4, 1989.

"You do think of your embryos," she said. "I bonded with mine. I talked to them. I told myself that they are only cells, but I had to talk to these cells that might be life."

She noted every procedure, every operation, hormone cycle and daily body temperature on a calendar in her neat cursive script—just as a new mother might compile the pages of a baby book.

Of the surgeries to remove the ripe eggs from her ovaries, she said, "All I really remember is someone yelling: 'Egg!'" During the embryo transfer itself, the door of the embryo laboratory was ajar. "It looked weird in there. All I could see were people in masks. I could hear this music coming out. It was sort of like the Twilight Zone." It was her only glimpse of the sanctum where her embryos were conceived or of the technicians who handled them.

All of them—patients and practitioners—were participants in an experiment that no federal regulatory authority had sanctioned, for which no public health agency had granted permission. The first embryo "hatching" procedure was conducted in Atlanta during May 1989, and the clinical trial continued into the following year. A medical-school review board would approve the experiment only after it was under way. The only federal board authorized to review such experiments had been disbanded for more than a decade. Three U.S. presidents—Jimmy Carter, Ronald Reagan, and George Bush—refused to revive it. Without it, no federally funded research on human embryos could be approved. With no funding, there was no control. Patients had no independent authority to guide them in evaluating new procedures. Scientists, especially those most concerned about improving success rates, were denied the funding to perform the systematic, controlled clinical trials needed to prove the safety of new techniques.

"The U.S. government is happier to fund research on animal reproduction to make better milk cows, or more prolific pigs, or chickens that lay more eggs," said Dr. Gary D. Hodgen, scientific director at the Jones Institute of Reproductive Medicine in Norfolk, Virginia.

Some congressmen protested a ban on research funding that, in effect, forced thousands of couples to exhaust their savings on relatively ineffective treatments. But Congress itself was no better. A Senate and House biomedical ethics board, obligated by law in part to consider the ethics of fetal research and the new technology of conception, stalled for five years. It held no hearings, issued no reports on the subject. Instead, it spent its time deadlocked over abortion.

Even for the most speculative procedures, public health officials and politicians found the creation of human embryos solely for research to be morally repugnant, as well as politically dangerous. Any experiment involving an early human embryo was to some degree controversial, as it involved material that was a potential human life. In the United States, that instinctive bias was the only safeguard against trivial or abusive experiments with human embryos. "Such a conservative posture, however, should not preclude truly innovative research directed toward important scientific or clinical advances," noted the ethics committee of the American Fertility Society.

Conventional medical ethics left only one acceptable avenue for researchers like Jacques Cohen: to use the woman as a living laboratory; to alter the human embryo, transfer it to its mother's womb, then hope the resulting child would be healthy and unharmed. Researchers had to experiment on what, if the cells survived the procedure and developed in the ensuing nine months, would one day become living children. There was no other ethical way to assess the effects on humans except through pregnancy. That was one point of view, but there were others. In 1990, British Parliament enacted a law stating that no embryo that has been used for research should be transferred to a woman.

Laboratory conception, including in vitro fertilization, had become the most powerful tool yet devised for the exploration of human reproduction. In the largest informal experiment in human biology ever conducted, more than 20,000 healthy IVF babies had been born around the world. Each squalling newborn, doctors said, was a testament to its safety. They spoke with the confidence of hindsight. In all its forms, laboratory conception had never been subject to a systematic, controlled trial in any country.

And how could it be? Few clinics followed the same protocols. They used different drugs, dosages, and culture techniques in an intuitive medical fugue on the creation theme. The resulting eggs differed subtly, not just from laboratory to laboratory, but from cycle to cycle in the same lab. Every laboratory handled the embryos in its own style. Many clinics were satisfied with a new technique after testing it on only 50 or 100 patients. Often, a single pregnancy would be deemed enough to validate an experiment. Medical authorities like Dr. Paul Lancaster, director of the National Perinatal Statistics Unit at the University of Sydney, warned that in order to detect the most subtle defects, a clinical trial would have to encompass thousands of pregnant women and the children they carried.

Cohen knew he was walking on dangerous ground. "Every time you do something new in this field, it is trouble," he said. "I am doing something here that is not reviewed. There is nothing forbidden in this country. There is just the fear—that one day I will do something detrimental. There are plenty of embryologists who could have done this thing, but fear kept them from doing it. Fear of what other people think kept them from doing it, not any law."

The stalemate left them all—couples who wanted a child, researchers who wanted to improve success rates, and the generations of children the couples had yet to conceive—in a clinical shadow where the line between therapeutic treatment and medical experiment was hard for anyone to see.

"We were willing to roll the dice with them," said patient Lisa Boone.

He was faceless—a man in a surgeon's mask who made life in a laboratory. At cocktail parties he would stand shyly by the wall and say, "I make babies for rich people," then grin wolfishly.

Working in a cramped third-floor laboratory barely the size of the average American bedroom, Jacques Cohen, thirty-eight, was one of the men guiding a revolution in human reproduction where life began outside the privacy of the womb in a succession of test tubes, Teflon-coated bowls called petri dishes, hot plates, cell freezers, and incubator ovens. He wanted no children of his own, yet spent his life helping others conceive them.

"A person wants children for selfish reasons," he would say. "Another person *doesn't* want children for selfish reasons. I know I am selfish."

Jacques Cohen was a man who thrived on the contradictions. He was twice married, twice divorced. He was a gifted sculptor, and a puppet master who built his own marionettes.

From distant cities, patients traveled to take advantage of his skills, yet the strangers whose eggs and sperm he manipulated so adroitly knew little of the procedures he performed in their service. They knew even less about him. It was their own doctor they thanked, the one who counseled them and heard their complaints, whose hand they shook, whose bill they paid.

If Cohen was a man who hated to talk directly to patients, he also was a man whose voice would rasp with emotion when he described their plight. He was a perfectionist in a field that demanded daily compromise, who found in the quarrelsome confines of an embryo laboratory something approaching peace.

By early 1989, the soft-spoken Dutch scientist had performed more than 4,000 in vitro fertilization cycles at clinics in New York, Atlanta, England, and Holland. Half a dozen clinics in the United States and Europe owed their success to his advice and supervision. He helped perfect embryo freezing. He was the first to achieve pregnancies from surgically altered human eggs and embryos. He served as the scientific midwife for hundreds of healthy children. "I read *Brave New World* and I liked it," Cohen said. He grinned. Freezing embryos, he once said in an expansive moment, was no harder than making good blueberry muffins. He hired his most reliable lab assistant based on her kitchen skills. But most of his peers found it difficult to match his success in achieving pregnancies or to keep pace with his appetite for innovation.

"There is a kind of fresh air around Jacques," said Alan Trounson, director of the Monash University Centre for Early Human Development in Melbourne, Australia. "He's good for the sport."

As a leading clinical embryologist, Cohen became a star in a world where scientists with doctorates traditionally were expected to take a back seat to doctors—to experiment with the mice and the baboons and leave the cash customers to the men and women with medical degrees. Cohen's growing expertise at micromanipulation only enhanced his reputation, for this skill was the key to a world of possibilities: microinjection of a single sperm, the repair of defective embryos, prenatal diagnosis of embryos, artificial twinning, embryo transplants, and genetic alterations of embryos.

"A good embryologist is valuable enough, but the people who are able to do these micromanipulation experiments are like gold. They are bought and sold on the international market," said Dr. Douglas M. Saunders, director of the IVF program at Royal North Shore Hospital in Sydney, Australia. "They are commodities like grain, oil, or precious metals."

In a field dominated by conservative gray suits and a starched bedside manner, Cohen was the perfect portrait of Eurochic. Presenting his research during the 1989 annual meeting of the American Fertility Society, Cohen stood on the podium in pleated black-balloon trousers, an embossed black-leather jacket, and black-leather high-tops. A black rubber tie with treads like a snow tire was held at his collar by a plain silver pin. Cohen's eyebrows were active punctuation marks as he smirked and glowered. The watch on his wrist had a black fly for a second hand: time flies.

Where Cohen often was a study in black and white—a kind of uptown Dutch Master—Henry Malter worked the entire spectrum. A quiet day found him in a lime green silk sport coat over a rust-blue-and-gold-colored camouflage shirt. His closely cropped red hair and beard were set off by a ponytail. From the lobe of his left ear dangled any one of an extensive earring collection—a tiny pair of silver handcuffs one day, a gold cross or a silver snake's coil the next. "This is one of my joke jackets," he said, cheerfully fingering a lapel.

The high style was, perhaps, their badge of scientific bravado. Several of Cohen's fellow embryologists admitted privately that they were uncomfortable experimenting with human embryos. It took too much nerve, too many futures at stake, too many political risks, they said. Two of the country's most respected embryologists tried human embryo work and then abandoned it. They slept more easily, they said, when they were cloning cow embryos or cleaving mouse eggs.

"If you were to think this is a potential human being, it would drive you crazy," Cohen said. "You know what I like? I like thawing embryos in the early morning or late at night when there's nobody around. There's something mystical about it. Just me and the embryos."

Jacques Cohen's laboratory in Atlanta was the last in a maze of rooms secured by combination locks that made up Reproductive Biology Associates (RBA), one of the more successful laboratory conception clinics in the United States. Dr. Hilton Kort, Dr. Joe Massey, and Dr. Carlene Elsner were partners in an infertility practice that sprawled across two floors of two brick office buildings near the superhighway that ringed the biggest boomtown in the old South. It was the only game in town. For all intents and purposes, the clinic held a monopoly on in vitro fertilization in a city of 2.8 million people. The couples it treated had a roughly one-in-four chance of becoming pregnant.

Massey and Kort were the founding partners. Kort, from South Africa, tailored, brisk, blond, had been a Ford Fellow at Yale University, then joined the Yale Medical School faculty before moving to Atlanta. Massey, a sleepy-eyed, affable

Emory University graduate, did his residency at the University of Pennsylvania Hospital in Philadelphia. But their practice traced its beginnings most directly to the Bourn Hall clinic in England, where Kort had observed Cambridge University Professor Robert G. Edwards and Patrick Steptoe, the two pioneers who created the world's first test-tube baby, at work, and to Melbourne, Australia, where Massey apprenticed for several weeks with two other IVF pioneers, Alan Trounson and Carl Wood. Kort and Massey had absorbed one important lesson: a doctor should keep out of the embryo laboratory.

"When we opened our clinic, we approached the problem from the perspective that the lab person was the key. We felt the lab person was critical," said Massey. "We could see there was going to be a lot of sinking and swimming. We did not want to fail."

In 1983, when test-tube babies were still the stuff of banner headlines, only a handful of embryologists had ever worked with human gametes and embryos. So Kort and Massey recruited the best basic scientist they could find. They persuaded Dr. Benjamin Brackett, then a leading authority on reproductive physiology at the University of Pennsylvania, to run their laboratory. The clinic opened in September 1983 and, within a month, announced its first pregnancy—Jeanine Catherine Caputo, born to Janet and Ray Caputo on Father's Day 1984. Her birth was so timely that Dan Rather announced her arrival on the CBS Evening News. Her face appeared on the front page of newspapers around the country. The clinic took the publicity to the bank, and in the six years following her birth, more than 1,000 couples sought out its services. The laboratory traffic would double and double again, then triple and quadruple. By 1990, the clinic had retrieved more than 14,000 human eggs, created more than 2,100 human embryos, and, from its plastic laboratory dishes, produced 275 babies.

Brackett, a distinguished embryologist whose work later earned him election to the National Academy of Sciences, resigned in 1984. He created the first test-tube lamb and the first test-tube calf. He created in vitro human babies for a year at RBA, but then gave it up because he found it too nerve-wracking and controversial. He became head of the Veterinary

College at the University of Georgia, where he sought ways to improve commercial cattle breeding.

Left without a scientific director, Kort remembered an overworked Dutch embryologist he had met over dinner at the prestigious Bourn Hall clinic in England—Jacques Cohen. "He had been through thousands of patients at Bourn Hall," said Massey. "We had done two hundred patients." Kort hired him. Within a year, Cohen doubled their clinic's birth rate. To pursue his research, he opened the Gamete and Embryo Research Laboratory at Emory University.

Dr. Elsner, an energetic woman with straight blond hair whose wry humor lines tugged at the corners of her mouth, joined the clinic in 1985. She had been a research fellow at the University of Pennsylvania. She started college when she was sixteen, graduated at nineteen, and went straight to the Medical College of Georgia. There were only two other women in the class. As part of her training, she did rounds at the public-health clinics in northern Florida. There, she recalled, the men wore IUD's in their hats like fishing lures and the women used red clay as a contraceptive plug. She took her partners—and herself—with liberal portions of salt.

"My patients tend not to be the real rich ones. The pushy, rich, demanding ones will be in Hilton's office. They all fall in love with him. Joe's patients tend to be the Southern belle magnolia types. I get the middle-management working couples. I also see patients who go off the wall with the other two. They see the ones who can't stand the sight of *my* face." She smiled, showing her teeth. "I have a husband at home who expects me to be a doctor's wife. I have two kids at home who expect me to be their mother. I tell them all I could be happy as a housewife. My husband doesn't believe me."

The clinic was in its own time zone. Its clocks ran by the menstrual cycle, a mainspring wound increasingly tight as the weeks wore on. The lab technicians started at dawn, panning with petri dishes for human eggs, and finished often after midnight, thawing embryos for transfer in the morning. During the 12 months of 1989, the clinic retrieved 1,890 eggs from 245 patients, created and transferred 725 fresh embryos, and made 69 women pregnant—a 28 percent pregnancy rate. Seventy-one babies were born. From the gray stainless-steel storage vats, they also thawed and transferred 195 frozen embryos into 104 women. Seventeen became pregnant. Any experiments were wedged, of necessity, into the clinical routine.

As hours turned into weeks, the embryologists felt as if they were trapped inside a cramped missile silo. There never seemed enough room. Someone was always in the way. In a lab space that seemed made up entirely of corners, doorways, and corridors, a single misstep, a sneeze, a jostled elbow, or a spill could mean disaster for an expectant couple's irreplaceable cells.

In empty moments—and between patient cycles there were hours of idle time—Cohen and his colleagues decorated the incubators, refrigerators, and embryo tanks with tabloid headlines, and the instruments with hand-lettered signs. The handle of one automatic pipette siphon warned: HAND-HELD NEUTRON BEAM WEAPON. POINT ONLY AT ENEMY. LETHAL RANGE—11 QUADRACS. It was free-form comic relief, a defensive reflex. It became a running commentary on the work—a collage of uneasy images culled from the scientific subconscious, murmurs of the id contained in the new idea:

"Docs Deliver Baby Frozen for 600 years."

"Space Alien Makes Girl, 7, Pregnant."

"Man Who Swallowed Whole Egg Hatches Chick in Stomach."

"Girl Gives Birth to a Chimpanzee in Tragic Sperm Bank Mix-up."

"Elvis Presley Sperm Bank: The King's Children Are Still Being Born."

And, taped to the office window: "I'm Pregnant with Satan's Baby."

Rubber snakes and plastic robots perched on the tops of computer monitors. In the hatch between the laboratory and the operating room sat a rubber bust of Ronald Reagan. An impatient embryologist would attract a nurse's attention by squeezing the president's head. The squeaks could be heard clearly even above the heavy breathing of the air conditioning and the wheezing embryo freezers.

On the refrigerator door someone had slapped a yellow bumper sticker: EGGS ANY TIME, ANY PLACE.

Working by remote control, Cohen reached for the embryo with the glass pipette. The embryo—four cells clustered inside a perfect translucent sphere—tumbled in the fluid. Steadying it with the pipette, he scraped away the stray cells clinging to the embryo. Then he eased the biopsy needle into the tough membrane that, like the shell around a chicken egg, encapsulated the budding cells.

With each infinitesimal movement of the needle, Cohen sidestepped the catch-22 of artificial conception: The procedure that enabled human life to begin in a laboratory dish also made it next to impossible for the resulting embryos to survive once they were transferred to the womb. Cohen and his colleagues suspected that, exposed outside the body, the embryo's protective outer membrane—called the zona pellucida—became so tough that the growing embryo could not escape. It died like a chick crushed inside its own shell.

Under the microscope, the embryo membrane was visible only as a translucent margin around the cluster of cells. Its two concentric layers served as more than just a shell. Without the zona membrane, conception could not take place. During fertilization itself, the sperm must touch it to become chemically activated. The zona membrane allowed only one sperm to reach the egg, and, in ways not completely understood, it eased the passage of the embryo through the fallopian tube. Laboratory observations suggested that as the embryo grew, the membrane should naturally thin, then open like a bud.

Even under the most natural conditions, however, most human embryos do not survive. Barely one-quarter develop into live-born infants. Most vanish during their journey through the fallopian tubes into the uterus during the short weeks between fertilization and actual implantation—before traditional diagnosis of pregnancy is even possible. Doctors estimated that about 60 percent of embryos never develop beyond a few cells. The lining of the uterus might not be receptive, or the embryos might be genetically flawed; they might have chromosomal abnormalities. In the laboratory, researchers were confident that they could put nature to shame. There, scientists could directly monitor the union of egg and sperm. There, they could be certain fertilization had occurred. They could assist defective sperm and ripen immature eggs. They could place viable embryos directly into the uterus.

The RBA clinic rose to prominence on a wave of new reproductive technology. The clinic's embryo laboratory produced the first documented pregnancies from frozen fertilized eggs, from human eggs surgically altered to enhance fertilization, and from embryos grown in an artificial womb of animal cells to improve their health. The laboratory produced 52 babies from surplus embryos that had been frozen in liquid nitrogen to avoid placing too many embryos in a woman's womb at any one time. In 1987, 39 U.S. clinics froze embryos for couples under treatment. In a single year, the number of U.S. clinics that offered the procedure and the number of embryos they placed in cold storage doubled. By 1988, 67 U.S. clinics froze more than 1,000 human embryos. In both years, however, just four clinics—RBA and three others—accounted for half of all the clinical pregnancies and half of all the delivered babies produced from frozen embryos.

Despite all the ministrations of medicine, however, laboratory embryos failed in even greater numbers. As the 1990s began, doctors and clinical embryologists around the world conducted about 75,000 IVF cycles every year—at a cost in the U.S. of up to $10,000 a cycle. Each cycle took 30 days. They regarded even a single pregnancy as an achievement.

Of those embryos transferred from the laboratory to the womb, fewer than one in every 10 embryos resulted in an established pregnancy; only one in 30 led to a live baby. In vitro fertilization produced twice as many spontaneous miscarriages; five times as many ectopic pregnancies; five times as many infants with spina bifida, a severe spinal-cord birth defect; and six times as many babies with an unusual heart defect called transposition. For in vitro fertilization, the rate of stillbirths and deaths in the first month of life was three times higher than normal. When doctors transferred the egg and sperm directly into the fallopian tube in a procedure called gamete intrafallopian transfer (GIFT), it was five times higher than normal.

More than one-third of all the human eggs obtained through in vitro fertilization had abnormal chromosomes. In all, only three out of every 100 human eggs doctors surgically retrieved from their patients' ovaries resulted in a viable live birth. Twelve years after the birth of the first test-tube baby, in a year when as many as 538 IVF clinics in 12 countries practiced laboratory conception, barely a handful could even come close to the natural unaided conception rate. The problem, many doctors agreed, was the laboratory process itself.

"There is enough evidence that there is a problem with embryos in IVF conditions," Cohen said. "We know that these embryos are not as good as natural-cycle embryos."

With quick flicks of the biopsy needle, Cohen stripped away the cells surrounding a second embryo. It was the brother or the sister of the first. He spun the embryo around, steadied it, and, in slow and deliberate motion, stabbed it with the needle. The pressure squeezed the embryo into a figure eight, as if it were trying to avoid the point. Then the needle suddenly slid through the membrane, and the embryo popped back into a sphere.

"There, it is harpooned," Cohen said.

He took a deep breath. The radio was playing Led Zeppelin. "This is a great lab," he said to himself, "but the music is terrible." Cohen twirled the embryo on the end of the needle. "Now we make a hole in it."

He gingerly moved the control knobs of the micromanipulator to make the pipette rub against the needle in a motion like that of a cricket rubbing its legs. The incision widened into a hole.

"The embryo will come out of the hole," Cohen said. "It clearly increases implantation. It goes from an average of six percent per embryo to an average of twenty-five percent. That is the most significant improvement I've ever heard of. Half a year ago, I would have said this is insane."

The operation itself took no more than five minutes. Cohen believed that for infertile couples seeking a child—and these couples almost always received multiple embryos from the laboratory—the micromanipulation of the embryo before implantation would double their chances for a pregnancy to an average of 50 percent—a rate better than any clinic in the world had achieved, and twice the natural conception rate among the healthiest young couples.

Anything that improved the ease and reliability of laboratory conception paved the way for its use in broader medical applications. It opened the way for scientists to intervene in the moment of conception and could also become a new tool for prenatal diagnosis—by enabling doctors to obtain the cells needed to detect inherited flaws months before conventional tests could reveal a problem. Embryologists like Cohen were creating tools for the correction of genetic diseases and chromosomal disorders in the embryo itself; what experts called the future of human reproduction. Eventually, laboratory conception could even become the key to the genetic engineering of children.

"The first time I saw egg and sperm under a microscope, it changed my life," Jacques Cohen said. Their microscopic union is, he said, the "big orgasm."

The youngest son of a Dutch Jewish middle-class merchant family, Cohen was born in 1951 in The Hague on the edge of the low country between the deltas, where the Netherlands feathers into Belgium and the North Sea. There, where only concrete surge barriers and earthen dikes hold back the sea's swell, the dividing line between land and water was an act of engineering. Cohen was raised in Maastricht, located at the southernmost tip of Holland, which, on the map of postwar Europe, welled like a teardrop into Belgium and Germany. Political and religious tides had given that border its shape. Born in the aftermath of the Nazi Occupation, Cohen remembers the family legacy of persecution.

"My parents survived the Holocaust by hiding," he said. "They were hiding in farms and apartments in little villages about four years. My mother and father both came from large families. Almost ninety percent died. They survived."

He was eighteen years old when he left home for the first time, to attend the university in Leyden. Biochemistry became his chosen study—the chemistry of living things. A notice on a university bulletin board started him on his career: FERTILIZATION OUTSIDE THE BODY, TO BE DONE IN MICE AND THE HUMAN. A doctoral student needed a research assistant. The ad, with its cryptic reference to human experiments, led him to an apprenticeship with the only experimental embryologist in Holland.

Cohen was dazzled. "When I saw the notice, I read it and thought: I will be able to manipulate the origin of life. Who would not want to do this? In fact, I was the only person who answered the ad," he said.

Cohen and other clinical embryologists like him found themselves caught in a kind of no-man's-land between basic science and clinical medicine. Licensing laws kept them from practicing their profession without the consent and supervision of a medical doctor. Regulatory restrictions prevented them from freely pursuing their research. His life's work was a discipline that drew equally from basic science and from clinical medicine, and that often received a measure of scorn from both.

For Cohen and his colleagues, the embryo was a moving point in the continuum of life. It was biology on a fast track, developing so quickly in its laboratory incubator that the technical vocabulary could barely keep pace: gamete, conceptus, zygote, four-cell, eight-cell, morula, blastocyst. In that thicket of terminology, researchers searched for the secure moral ground on which to conduct their work. If the public objected to experiments with human embryos, researchers would work on the pre-embryo. If a legislature declared that life began at conception, the researchers would redefine conception.

Cohen approached his work with a fundamental gravity. He was not, he said, a religious man. He was an atheist. The respect he accorded the embryo was the respect he believed all life deserved. "When the law starts to define the onset of life, it is a joke. Life doesn't stop and then start again. It is a continuum. The egg and sperm go together and make an embryo. That embryo in part becomes a fetus supported by the embryonic tissue and the placenta. Then you have birth and a new individual who can support himself after a while. That same individual carries the genome, the set of genes inherited from both parents, and has it already in the reproductive organs." Life was a circle with no end and no beginning. Each woman's ovary contained half a million eggs that developed in the womb before she herself was born. "I don't know where life starts. I think it started three billion years ago with Genesis."

Other groups struggled with their own definition of human life. The argument took the abortion debate into a moment before there even was a fetus to protect, when there were only a few cells with the potential of becoming human. By 1990, scores of religious, legislative, and professional organizations had published reports on the status of the embryo and the new technology. The answers they arrived at—after reams of expert testimony, parliamentary points of order, and thoughtful deliberation—did little to settle the question.

An embryo was not a person, they all agreed. But, then, just what was it? The Vatican ruled that any human being was to be respected and treated as a person "from the moment of conception." Church authorities didn't want any hair-splitting about terminology. "No moral distinction is considered between zygotes, pre-embryos, embryos, or fetuses," church authorities said. By law in Minnesota, an embryo was considered alive enough to be a victim of criminal homicide, and one man who killed his girlfriend went on trial for murdering one. Neither of them had known she was pregnant. To a state judge in Tennessee, embryos were "living children." In Louisiana an embryo was a disembodied courtroom presence: As a matter of state law since 1986, an embryo could sue and be sued. To the Louisiana legislature, at least, the situation was clear; the laboratory embryo was neither living child nor adult, but potential litigant.

"We are constantly trying to apply distinctions which pertain in ordinary life but which do not actually apply in a particular respect," said the Archbishop of York in the British House of Lords. "For example, lawyers try to put everything in one of two baskets—it is either a person or a thing. However, there are entities which are neither persons nor things. What we are referring to in the case of a conceptus is an organism of human origin which, given the right conditions, has the potential to develop and may become a full human person."

To the men and women whose gametes produced it, the embryo embodied dreams of parenthood; a powerful symbol of hope clothed in the illusion of flesh. The physical procedures that produced them—with its needles, operating rooms, and weeks of discomfort—was a parental rite of passage that became its own labor of delivery. There was a piece of themselves in the world, growing in a culture dish or frozen in a vat. Even as they braced themselves for failure, they often bonded with the embryos in a dress rehearsal for pregnancy.

The laboratory rites made the life of the cells a public ceremony that extended the idea of the developing child into the moment before its genetic structure had even fused—before it was even by the most scientific standard anything resembling a unique individual. It implanted the embryos in the mind, long before they ever reached the womb, before they could appear as echoes on an ultrasound screen, before they could quicken, kick, and make themselves known.

Couples fretted over the quality of their infinitesimal progeny as anxiously as any new parent. They listened as intently to the doctor's diagnosis. "These are beautiful embryos, the best I've ever seen," Dr. Hilton Kort would tell them. Consciously or not, the doctors spoke in the language of living infants. In the operating room at the Jones Institute of Reproductive Medicine in Norfolk, Dr. Michael Edelstein handed his patient the petri dish in which her embryos had been conceived. "Here is your baby's first crib," he said proudly.

Cohen had been brooding over the idea of embryo surgery since the spring of 1984. He had thawed two frozen embryos that year at Bourn Hall and, with embryologist Carole Fehilly, put a hole in both with a hypodermic needle to make an artificial gap in the zona membranes. Neither embryo survived and they abandoned the experiment. "We got scared," Cohen said. Five years later, Cohen plucked an idea from a scientific journal that made him revive it.

In the *Journal of Experimental Zoology*, researchers Jon Gordon and Beth Talansky at The Mount Sinai Medical Center in New York City showed that it was possible to dissolve a hole in the membrane around a mouse egg and open a path for sperm to enter more easily. The technique, which they called zona-drilling, promised to improve dramatically the treatment of male infertility by enabling weak sperm to penetrate the egg. They did to mouse eggs what Cohen and Fehilly tried to do to human embryos.

Sitting in Cohen's kitchen, Beth Talansky, her face surrounded by a thick corona of stylishly unruly brown hair, explained: "We decided to look at things from the approach of manipulating the egg. The simplest approach seemed to be, instead of poking around inside it too much, to just drill a little opening in the zona to see if we could facilitate sperm entry that way. It was very simple. The best ideas are simple, right?" Talansky and Gordon found that they could increase the number of fertilized mouse eggs by about 75 percent, and also showed that the eggs produced normal offspring. Cohen was impressed.

If the process worked in mice, however, it proved almost impossible to get the zona-drilling technique to work with humans. Cohen tried, failed, failed again. To perfect the techniques of micromanipulation, embryologists had mounted a new wave of scientific assaults on the human egg. They drilled it. They etched it with acid. They ripped its membranes with microscopic glass hooks. They pushed it around with laser beams. Cohen remembered the hypodermic needle and the embryo-hatching experiment at Bourn Hall. Perhaps he could adapt that technique to the human egg. Instead of etching a hole with acid, he slit the egg with a glass needle.

Where other clinics in the United States and abroad failed, Cohen and Henry Malter succeeded. By the end of 1989, six babies had been born to couples whose eggs had been surgically opened. Four of the six children were twins. And 47 more women were pregnant. In all, Malter and Cohen had operated on 400 eggs. All but 16 survived. The surgery doubled the fertilization rate among infertile men. Preliminary results indicated it also doubled the pregnancy rate. Immediately it became part of RBA's clinical routine. Other clinics were skeptical. Partial zona dissection—PZD, as Cohen dubbed the variation—was largely dependent on the skill of the person performing the surgery. Forging the microtools was an art in itself.

There were problems. Many of the resulting embryos were genetically abnormal because more than one sperm slipped through the hole in the membrane; they had to be discarded. If too many sperm penetrated the egg, it died.

But, overall, more eggs became fertilized and, surprisingly, more of the resulting embryos implanted in the women's wombs. The reason, Cohen believed, had to be the hole.

Jacques Cohen checked the two embryos under the microscope again. They had survived the micromanipulation nicely and were ready to be placed in the mother's womb.

It was still an August Sunday morning in Atlanta. Only an hour had passed. The altered embryo waited with two others in a shallow plastic dish. The California couple had finished their coffee and driven from their nearby hotel. They waited with Dr. Elsner in the transfer room. Cohen, his expression hidden now behind a surgical mask, bent over a microscope wreathed in a green fluorescent glow. A flute concerto had replaced Led Zeppelin on the portable radio.

Working with quick, deft movements, he rotated the dish until he could see the couple's name etched on its bottom. He checked the name against his records. He slid the dish under a second microscope connected to a camera and snapped a time-stamped Polaroid photograph of the embryos.

Back now at the first microscope, he loaded the couple's three embryos into a pliable plastic catheter and, holding it aloft like an acolyte with an altar candle, padded quickly into the next room.

There the only light was the glow from the high-powered physician's headlamp Elsner wore. The woman rested back on a wheeled gurney waiting to receive the embryos. A sheet was draped across her knees. Her husband stood at her side, a hand on her shoulder.

Elsner lifted the sheet and threaded the catheter into the woman's uterus. No one spoke or seemed to breathe. When it was positioned, Cohen leaned forward and injected the embryos, pushing the plunger gently while Elsner held the catheter steady.

In a second, it was done.

"Who's got the picture?" said Elsner. The Polaroid photograph of the embryos was placed into the patient's hands. For a moment she was confused, uncertain of what she held and what it meant. Then she recognized them. The woman beamed, pressing the Polaroid to her breast. She knew it might be the only picture of her children she ever saw.

The embryos were now on their own. It would be weeks before anyone would know if they had survived and a pregnancy had officially begun. In the interim, only Cohen knew that he had altered the embryos in the woman's womb. In accordance with the standard terms of a controlled, blind trial, the couple would not be told whether the operation had been performed until after the results of the pregnancy tests were known.

"I have done something that works, but I don't know how," Cohen said. "I still have a few doubts about making a hole in the embryo, about what it does."

The hole in the barrier let the embryo out, but it also might let the attack cells of the body's immune system in. The immune system cells are attracted by certain chemical signals; a biochemical friend-or-foe system that is the body's main defense against disease. If the immune cells do not register the proper signal from a cell, they are programmed to attack it. They might sniff the strange embryo through the artificial opening, like junkyard dogs scenting a burglar coming through a hole in the fence.

If the woman became pregnant, the odds were higher that she would bear twins, or even triplets. As the embryo "hatched" through the hole that Cohen had made, there was a chance it could be squeezed and pinched off or simply disintegrate. Cohen called this the "Pac-Man effect." If enough of the embryo were caught as it emerged, it could split into pieces large enough to become identical twins. The second infant would be a by-product of surgery, an artificial twin produced through accidental cloning of the embryo. If the hole was too big, the embryo could fall out and hatch too soon. Cohen and his colleagues also worried that if the developing embryo were to be caught half in and half out of the hole in the zona, it would grow into Siamese twins joined at the head, or shoulder or hip. It had never happened, but they worried that it might. There was no shortage of concerns, and no way to lay them to rest.

Cohen would have to wait. It was ironic: Since their moment of conception, the embryos had been available for his inspection under the microscope. Now they were inaccessible. No matter what happened to them, Cohen would never be sure whether he had helped or hindered their development; he could only make an educated guess. The mystery had reasserted itself.

By the fall of 1989, Jacques Cohen's team had operated on 115 embryos in three separate clinical trials. All 115 survived the procedure and half the women in the experiment became clinically pregnant. But even before the first child was born or the first research paper published, the results were transmitted on the informal grapevine that links infertile couples in clinic waiting rooms across the country. Joe Massey of Reproductive Biology Associates and Zev Rosenwaks of Cornell spread the word at clinical conferences.

At Reproductive Biology Associates, women threatened to cancel treatment unless their embryos were "hatched" by Cohen's team. "The patients are clamoring for it," said Massey. The doctors agreed to offer it to all who asked. At Cornell, Cohen insisted they still treat the procedure as experimental, but he offered it as widely as possible to patients.

Still the doctors and the embryologists hesitated. There was the possibility that the surgery was only producing a greater number of phantom pregnancies—biochemical pregnancies that register on the standard pregnancy tests but that only end in miscarriage. The lab staff and the doctors conferred throughout December, torn between conducting additional, limited trials or offering the technique as part of the standard clinical, therapeutic routine. "As a scientist, I'm not sure if we really should be doing hatching on everyone yet," said Michael

Tucker, the senior embryologist at Reproductive Biology Associates. "But as someone who is trying to get people pregnant, I say we have to go ahead. You are always torn between the two."

The results were still unclear, still hard to interpret. They needed to know more. They would begin another clinical trial. Like the expectant parents, they needed to see the babies born.

2

Waiting Rooms

The wooden bench was as hard and cold as a Pentecostal Church pew. Its slats left creases in the damp suit jackets of the three husbands who sat on it, waiting between the red bags of medical waste and a row of battered lockers on the eighth floor of New York Hospital. They pulled their legs in to avoid getting their wingtips scuffed by the nurses and doctors who burst through the swinging double doors like carnival bumper cars.

The three men were tense. It showed in their shoulders and in the way they avoided conversation. One bowed his head in the pages of a paperback techno-thriller. The other two stared at the beige door of Room M-803—a converted broom closet, really—where, in a moment, each would be expected to produce a sperm sample quickly and efficiently. The nurses call it the Jack Room.

Outside, at the corner of East Seventieth Street and York Avenue, it was a Manhattan morning rush hour. Traffic was snarled. The September sky was the color of wet pavement. Pedestrians leaned their umbrellas into the wind and rain. Inside, by the operating room and embryo laboratory of the Cornell Center for Reproductive Medicine, the three men waited to make babies. The hall was as close as they were allowed. They were not welcome inside the embryo laboratory. They were not allowed to accompany their wives into the operating room.

There, the doctors had started to collect eggs from the first patient of the day with an ultrasound probe. As the morning progressed, other women would take her place. The embryologists, like air-traffic controllers, were set to usher the men in and out of the small bathroom to get each fresh sperm specimen as quickly as possible. In the andrology laboratory next door, a technician would label it, wash it, analyze it, spin it in a centrifuge, and, at the proper moment late that evening, use it to fertilize the woman's eggs. At that moment of consummation, both husband and wife would be far away, most likely asleep in their own bed.

The first man was late, delayed by the rain. The schedule started to slide. Minutes ticked away. One man paged deeper into his book; the other two shifted in their seats and stared at the bathroom door. Lab technician Adrienne McVicker finally beckoned to the next man on the list. He put down his book, accepted the specimen cup, and listened glumly to the instructions. "If you could put your name on it," she told him. A doctor brushed past them both in the hallway. Two nurses conferred by the lockers.

Suddenly, the double doors whipped open and, in a swirl of dripping umbrella and blurted apologies, the first man made his appearance. He saw McVicker. "I'm so sorry," he said. "I was caught in traffic." He shook the umbrella.

With hardly a word, she retrieved the specimen cup and handed it to the new arrival. In an instant, he had disappeared behind the beige-metal door while the other man resumed his seat and his place in the paperback.

"Finally," McVicker said briskly as she walked back into the embryo laboratory and closed the door, "we've got this sperm wagon moving."

Seated at a lab bench, senior embryologist Mina Alikani quickly looked up, smiled fleetingly, then focused her almond eyes again through the microscope in front of her. Systematically, she checked the human eggs stored overnight in the incubator to see how many had actually fertilized. She quickly found the first.

The microscope revealed a single, enormous translucent cell as imperfectly round as a hand-compacted snowball. During the night, a single sperm cell had pushed its way through the protein membrane surrounding the egg and spilled its contents inside. As it entered, the one sperm transformed the chemistry of the membrane, turning it into an impenetrable barrier blocking any straggling sperm cells.

Inside the gelatinous sphere, two smaller circles were barely visible. One contained the chromosomes from the mother; the other the father's genetic inheritance. They had not yet merged. It would be hours before they would completely fuse. The egg was less than one-tenth of a millimeter long. It weighed less than two milligrams. Under magnification, the fertilized egg glistened in its plastic dish like a seed pearl.

"She is pregnant," said Alikani, looking very pleased. "Well, she is pregnant in a dish, I suppose."

She carefully replaced the dish in the incubator and shut the door. Now the incubator was pregnant. In 24 hours, a doctor would move the new embryo into the prospective mother's womb. To reach that point, the couple had spent between $5,000 and $10,000.

Alikani and McVicker moved with practiced grace. There were five more egg retrievals, five inseminations, and two embryo transfers on the schedule before lunchtime; 20 couples scheduled that week; about 600 couples that year. For them, it would take months, sometimes years, to reach the point where someone could proudly say: *Pregnant in a dish.*

As the 1990s began, an entire generation of men and women camped at the threshold of conception; unable to conceive a child of their own and not yet willing to concede defeat.

The activity at the Cornell clinic was mirrored, with only minor variations, in the waiting rooms and hallways of hundreds of conception clinics like RBA in Atlanta and around the world. A half-dozen had opened in New York City alone. There were 13 within a day's drive of Washington, D.C., and

11 in the Los Angeles area. Congressional investigators counted 160. The U.S. General Accounting Office found 200. There were 38 clinics in England, 24 in Australia. There were dozens more in Europe, Africa, and Japan. There was at least one mammoth state-run clinic in Moscow, another in Leningrad. There were 528 in a dozen countries. No one had any idea how many there were worldwide.

Where were all the patients coming from? Throughout Western Europe, birth rates tumbled. Overall, the incidence of infertility in the United States had remained a constant for 20 years. Some experts suggested that between 1962 and 1988, the infertility rate, like the national birth rate, had declined slightly. Even so, the National Center for Health Statistics found in 1990 that, in terms of sheer numbers, more people than ever before were unable to conceive, a total of 4.9 million women between the ages of fifteen and forty-four years old in 1988 alone.

A closer look showed that, while the overall percentage of infertile men and women may have dropped, the burden of childlessness had shifted. Among the youngest couples—those between twenty and twenty-four years old—the incidence of infertility had tripled. Some placed the overall number as high as 15 percent of the population of childbearing age. "That's ten million to twelve million people," said Barbara Eck Manning, the former Boston nurse who founded Resolve, an infertility support group with chapters in 50 U.S. cities. "I believe we will see an epidemic of infertility in the coming decade."

Some experts, however, argued that an epidemic of medical marketing was equally responsible for the dramatic increases. In 1987, only half the country's infertile couples sought a doctor's help to conceive. To reach the others, medical marketing executives worked overtime. The number of office visits to infertility specialists tripled. Marketing campaigns that only a few years before attempted to exploit sex and the single consumer now celebrated the commercial joys of family and parenthood. The October 20, 1990, issue of *Time* magazine was typical. On its inside back cover, an automobile advertisement asked the reader: IS SOMETHING INSIDE YOU TELLING YOU TO

BUY A VOLVO? The headline, accompanied by a tiny photograph of a Volvo station wagon, was superimposed over a full-page ultrasound image of a fetus in the womb.

The couples were caught up in a national spawning season that rivaled the baby boom of the 1950s. In 1989, a year when demographers predicted that the national birth rate would fall, more children were born in the United States than in any other year since the last baby boom crested in 1964. The couples all shared the same vision of the American dream: If they worked hard enough, if they saved enough, if they followed the proper medical procedures, charted their temperatures, and had regular sex, they would have a child. More people became parents for the first time in 1987—the most recent year for which numbers were available—than at any other time in U.S. history. The number of the newborn edged toward 4 million a year.

Couples who postponed childbearing were in the last leg of their race with age. As the 1990s began, more older women were having children than ever before. Women who were "thirty-something" accounted for one-third of all U.S. births, compared to one-fifth only 10 years before. The number of women who were having their first child in their thirties had quadrupled between 1970 and 1986. The percentage of childless wives in their early thirties who said they were still planning to have children had almost doubled since 1975.

Half the women in the United States over twenty-five were still waiting to conceive, a portion unmatched since the depths of the Great Depression. Those women and their partners filled the waiting rooms of IVF clinics. Each waiting room offered a port of entry into the same foreign country:

At Reproductive Biology Associates in Atlanta, the couples parked on white sofas in a waiting room decorated with abstract paintings, and thumbed through copies of *Art in America* and *Vanity Fair*. A woman in a tangerine-colored cable-knit sweater talked in a hushed voice about pregnancy rates and hormone surges to the gray-haired, blue-eyed woman sitting next to her. They exchanged notes about sperm donors and culture mediums.

At the Jones Institute of Reproductive Medicine in Norfolk, Virginia, they waited in blue armchairs under color photographs of petri dishes and human eggs. Newcomers stared at the brass plaque near the receptionist. It listed, in chronological order, the birth dates of 500 babies conceived at the clinic. "There, my baby is number two hundred seventy-six," said Carolyn Abernethy, pointing to the date on the plaque: February 9, 1987. When she was twenty-two years old, a doctor told Abernethy she could never have a child. Now she was forty and, thanks to a Norfolk embryologist, already had one son. She had returned to conceive a second.

At the IVF Australia Clinic in Port Chester, New York, women waited under five enormous photographs of couples playing with newborn infants. The clinic's unusual name reflected its corporate ties to the Australian scientists who pioneered many of the IVF procedures. Hand-lettered messages on a bulletin board reached out to the other strangers in the room: ANYONE IN THE BENSONHURST BKLYN AREA WHO WOULD LIKE TO TALK. PLEASE CALL MARLENE* AND TOM.* ANYONE IN L.I. WHO WOULD LIKE TO TALK, CALL CAROLINE* AND JEROME.* COUPLE WITH SECONDARY INFERTILITY CYCLING WITH IVF AUSTRALIA WOULD LIKE TO TALK WITH PERSONS WHO CAN RELATE. BELINDA* AND MARTY.*

At the fashionable Harley Street headquarters of the Hallam Medical Centre in London, the waiting couples sipped tea from flowered bone-china cups in a formal front parlor papered in pale blue silk. The ceiling was inlaid with frescoes of scenes from Greek and Roman mythology. Clusters of pink gladiolus flanked the doors. In the basement operating room, one man sat on a stool by his wife's left shoulder as the doctor harvested her eggs. The man squeezed her hand under the sheet.

At the Infertility Medical Centre at Epworth Hospital in Melbourne, Australia, the expectant couples sat in double rows of spartan metal armchairs. A poster on the wall declaimed: SEMEN DONORS REQUIRED IN ALL SHAPES AND SIZES. Every year, the Epworth clinic treated about 1,200 couples. At the end of a long, dark corridor, patient counselor Louise Bowen waited in her office doorway for the next couple. "What we are facing

here is the harsh reality that most of them are going to fail,"
she said. It was what the scientists faced everywhere.

Every clinic was an Olympus for a local fertility god. Some
were run by medical pioneers; others by obstetricians who,
driven by fears of malpractice litigation, abandoned delivering
babies for the more profitable pursuit of treating the married
couples who could not conceive them. Their embryo incubators
housed secrets, hopes, and fears, including those of the staff:
the embryologist obsessed with his declining sperm count; the
doctor who gave his technicians the day off so that no one
would know he was impregnating his wife by in vitro fertilization; the embryologist who tried to persuade his married
lover to donate her eggs, so that a surrogate mother could
bear their clandestine child.

The clinics were tightly knit and fiercely competitive. They
jockeyed for professional prestige and a place in the footnotes
of medical history. Some were slippery about it, studiously
vague about their success rates, or, in a few cases, blatantly
fraudulent. There was more at stake than a pecking order:
Analysts in 1988 estimated the U.S. infertility market at $2.4
billion a year. They predicted that laboratory conception itself
would generate $430 million a year. But how to fill the waiting
rooms with customers? There was word of mouth, of course;
every new baby was a living billboard for the clinic that produced it. Each clinic had its stud book in the waiting room—
a kind of Sears catalogue of conception, bulging with photographs of infants conceived in the clinic laboratory. It could
be a powerful sales tool.

"I walked into the office and there were all these baby pictures. I stopped short," said one prospective patient. "All of
a sudden I couldn't see anything, I couldn't hear anything.
Like someone just hit me with a baseball bat."

But preeminent professional standing was the best advertising a clinic could have. It earned its doctors invitations to
talk shows and put them before congressional panels as expert
witnesses. The leading researchers could hold educational
seminars for other doctors, and thereby expand their pool of
referring physicians. Such a reputation took more than a public

relations consultant; it required a substantial and sincere investment in research. New medical journals, peer review boards, and professional societies were organized to channel the resulting flood of research papers.

For more than a decade, the Jones Institute of Reproductive Medicine in Norfolk had reigned supreme as the leading infertility clinic in the United States. Dr. Howard W. Jones, Jr., and Dr. Georgeanna Jones were genuine pioneers, responsible for the first child conceived in an American laboratory. Doctors in England had conceived the world's first, doctors in Australia the world's second. In the United States, however, third place finished first.

All of it was refugee research, stalled by ethics deliberations in some countries, public outrage in others. It was research that flourished best out of the public eye. Suppressed in America, France, and Holland, it raced ahead in England. It flourished in Australia, then became mired in parliamentary politics. The research focus moved to the United States, then to Asia, and again to England, shifting from place to place like the hidden pea in a shell game. When each breakthrough came, it always seemed to be the work of a laboratory far from the center of things.

"There was an international IVF mafia," said Howard Jones in Norfolk. He took down a photograph from his office bookshelf. In it, a dozen smiling men and women gathered around a garden bench on the lawn of an English manor house. The year was 1982. It might have been a yearbook photograph of a prep-school headmaster and his faculty. Jones kept it as a souvenir of creation, a portrait of the cast that taught the world to master human conception. The same picture is thumbtacked to the wall in Alan Trounson's office in Melbourne, Australia. He stood in bell-bottomed jeans, boyish and barrel-chested, in the photo's back row. The same photo also hung in a village nine miles west of Cambridge, England, in a room occupied by Cambridge University Professor Robert G. Edwards. He sat on the bench at the center of the photograph, his shaggy hair curling over his collar. Edwards was the first to conceive a child outside the human body. "Oh, you mean God," one of his apprentices would later say when Edwards's name was mentioned.

Between 1971 and 1978, Edwards and his research partner, gynecologist Patrick Steptoe, experimented with 80 women, trying to impregnate them with laboratory embryos. None became pregnant. The chances of success were remote in any species. Only 200 rabbits conceived outside the body had been born; about 200 mice; fewer than 50 rats. When they finally succeeded in 1978 it took even the newly expectant mother by surprise. Only then did she realize she was going to give birth to the world's first test-tube baby. "I don't remember Mr. Steptoe ever saying whether his method of producing babies had ever worked and I certainly didn't ask," recalled Lesley Brown in her account of the experience. "I just imagined that hundreds of children had already been born through being conceived outside their mothers' wombs."

It took 18 years from the moment Edwards first conceived a human embryo outside the womb until he was able to bring a fetus full-term. The obstacles he and Steptoe faced were only partly technical. As they struggled to achieve their first test-tube pregnancy, members of Parliament demanded that the government investigate their experiments. The British Medical Research Council, voicing "serious doubts about the ethical aspects of the proposed investigations in humans," spurned their requests for research funding. Even the Ford Foundation, which had been a major underwriter of research into human reproduction, cut off its direct funding. The foundation was more interested in work to curb population growth, its officials explained. The two beleaguered pioneers financed their work with Steptoe's earnings from legal abortions.

With surprising speed, other researchers transformed the major surgery of egg retrieval into an outpatient procedure. They broadened the applications of laboratory conception with new techniques that turned almost all women and men into potential clients. Never had scientists and doctors so artfully bypassed the barriers thrown up by nature or disease to bar the creation of human life.

Within a decade, scientists learned to pinpoint and extract

a single human egg from its ovary, then, with synthetic hormones, to take charge of women's menstrual cycles to produce eggs on demand. They learned to shift embryos from one woman to the next. They learned to determine an embryo's sex and caught their first glimpses of the genes that controlled its development. Molecular biologists held out the promise that within a decade or more, they could consciously tailor an embryo's genetic structure. Age, infertility, virginity, and menopause were no longer bars to pregnancy.

In private clinics, scientists soon sought ways to ripen artificially the thousands of primordial human egg cells stored from birth in a woman's ovaries—each no larger than a few thousandths of an inch in size. In 1989, doctors at Cha Women's Hospital in Seoul, Korea, extracted undeveloped egg cells from a human ovary, grew them in the laboratory without any artificial hormones, and successfully fertilized them. They put the resulting embryos in the uterus of a twenty-eight-year-old volunteer who, by the time the doctors made their experiment public, had given birth to triplets. The research raised the possibility that surgeons could harvest an entire ovary, grow the egg cells it contained in dishes like tomatoes in a hydroponic garden, and harvest hundreds of human eggs at once. The Korean team created a primitive but workable artificial ovary. They produced three babies—and not a ripple in the headlines.

But almost a decade earlier, when Howard and Georgeanna Jones attempted to create the first in vitro baby in the United States, they faced hostile committee hearings in the Virginia General Assembly. Crowds of pro-life demonstrators protested the wastage of human embryos, and U.S. Senator Orin Hatch, R-Utah, threatened a congressional investigation. Success, however, silenced the critics. The aging husband-and-wife medical team did in their retirement years what doctors at the peak of their careers in Australia and England could not—they made laboratory conception respectable. In their hands, its practice became an exercise in the highest professional responsibility. They set the gold standard; then they went one step further. They established the largest U.S. research institute devoted to clinical human reproduction, with 125 scientists, doctors, technicians, and nurses. Their stud book ran to 10 volumes.

On their lobby wall hung an endorsement unique in the annals of American medicine: "The Norfolk group is the acknowledged leader in in vitro fertilization and embryo transfer in the United States. These scientists' superior results and inquisitive bent, coupled with the fact that theirs is the unit that has been active the longest in this country, make their leadership an uncontested fact." The quote came from the April 9, 1987, issue of *The New England Journal of Medicine*—a publication considered so authoritative that in medical matters it passed for the voice of God.

In 1985, the Jones Institute had a backlog of 10,000 couples seeking the laboratory's help in conceiving a child. But the clinic quickly lost its U.S. monopoly and, as patients scattered to newer clinics, its waiting list shrank to a few hundred. By 1990, there was no waiting at all. Patients were more aggressive, more demanding, harder to satisfy. The Jones Institute got only the hardest, most intractable—and often most disappointing—cases. The research spotlight had shifted. Howard and Georgeanna Jones had no plans to retire, but, as they entered their eighties with undiminished vigor, their colleagues at the clinic were braced for an inevitable change in leadership.

So were their competitors. At New York Hospital and Cornell Medical Center, administrators marshaled their resources to edge the Norfolk clinic from its throne. They were prepared to spend millions to turn the Cornell Center for Reproductive Medicine into one of the nation's leading infertility research centers.

It was to be a kind of palace coup organized, oddly enough, by the crown prince. Cornell persuaded Norfolk's longstanding medical director, Dr. Sev Rosenwaks, to lead its effort. In the fall of 1988, Rosenwaks, a leading authority on human reproduction, left his mentors and the institute that bore their name. As his first move at Cornell, Rosenwaks set about recruiting Jacques Cohen in Atlanta. Throughout early 1989, he promised Cohen and Malter a place on the Cornell faculty, new laboratories, extra staff, the newest equipment, and, of course, a bigger salary. The entire package would cost about $4.5 million.

The two women were sisters of a sort—the soft-spoken, wan wallflower and the voluble Viking in a Yukon pullover and hiking shorts. Both were brilliant, stubborn, determined to succeed. One was a doctor; the other owned her own company. And in September 1989, they found themselves sitting at opposite ends of the waiting room at the Jones Institute in Norfolk.

Both had been permanently scarred by defective birth-control devices—their IUD's. Both had miscarried repeatedly. Both had suffered through ectopic pregnancies and both were infertile. Yet both had a child.

Carolyn Abernethy conceived her son with the help of the doctors at Norfolk. She was still a plaintiff in court over the damage caused by her Dalkon Shield IUD. Mara Molin* had adopted a baby after trying and failing in a dozen IVF attempts at Norfolk and other hospitals. They both had come to Norfolk to make a second child. At forty, both women faced a 50 percent higher chance of spontaneous miscarriage.

"If there is hope, it's just very hard for me to give it up. You just keep going until it's too late by age, or until other people give up on you," Mara Molin said. After science failed her a dozen times, she briefly gave up on herself. Only her adopted child gave her the strength to continue. "She's been very healing for me. She makes me want to have more children."

She waited to ovulate under the influence of drugs designed to push her ovaries into overdrive and force production of a dozen or more eggs at once. Carolyn Abernethy waited for her frozen embryos to thaw, to see how many would survive their sojourn in suspended animation. She had frozen embryos in storage up and down the East Coast. Her efforts to conceive so far had cost $100,000, she said. Most of it had come out of her own pocket. The remainder was paid by her insurance company.

For these women, the only thing worse than failing to become pregnant was to be kept from trying. Both Abernethy and Molin were part of an afternoon tide that drifted into the waiting room at Norfolk's Hofheimer Hall—infertile women checking in for blood tests and hormone shots. They had tried and failed elsewhere. They had come to the Jones Institute in Norfolk because they were convinced it was the best. The waiting room would become their second home.

If there was a growing epidemic of infertility in the United States, there was no shortage of things to blame it on. Endometriosis and ovarian cysts affected thousands of women. Tobacco contributed to infertility. Aspirin inhibited a woman's ability to ovulate. Too much exercise could contribute. The antihistamines that many people took to control their hay fever could impair sperm; so did hot baths and tight underwear. Caffeine affected the fertility of men and women. Stress, pollution, pesticides—there was a lengthy litany.

For many women like Abernethy and Molin, birth control had crippled their ability to conceive. Plastic interuterine devices (IUD's) like the Dalkon Shield tripled the risk of pelvic infections and doubled the risk of infertility. Experts estimated that 8.6 million American women had used the loops of plastic, and at least 88,000 of them might be unable to have children as a result. The manufacturer, A. H. Robins Co., was besieged with so many lawsuits that it sought refuge in bankruptcy, leaving behind a $2.5 billion trust fund to settle 300,000 claims from injured women in 80 countries. G. D. Searle Co., which manufactured an IUD called the Copper-7 sold to about 10 million women, was hit with 1,000 lawsuits. The Searle family sold the company.

Thousands of other women couldn't conceive due to a drug their mothers had taken during pregnancy to prevent miscarriage. The daughters of women who were prescribed a powerful synthetic hormone called Diethylstilbestrol (DES) inherited a high risk of infertility, ectopic pregnancies, and cancer. The sons also inherited infertility problems. Evidence emerged in 1990 that DES may have afflicted their granddaughters, as well. About 267 companies made the drug; virtually all of them were being sued.

Almost half the time, it was the men who could not make a baby. Sperm counts had dropped by more than half in 30 years, and low sperm count was the primary reason for male infertility. Some studies showed that male sperm counts dropped from an average of 200 million sperm cells per milliliter in the 1930s to less than 70 million in many cases during the 1980s.

Researchers tried and failed to link infertility to abortion, while the popular press often blamed childlessness on the changing status of women—depicting infertility as a biological penalty for social change. They ignored the effects of inflation and cost-of-living increases that made two-career couples as much a matter of economic necessity as of equality and women's rights.

In large part, infertility was a preventable plague. For many couples, their inability to conceive was the result of sexually transmitted diseases so prevalent in the United States that only the common cold and influenza were more widespread. Yet, among women, the diseases were so rarely detected or diagnosed that, untreated, they caused about 125,000 new cases of infertility every year.

Sexually transmitted diseases struck most heavily among young women twenty-four years old or less—those entering their peak childbearing years. Because they often showed no symptoms, many women had been permanently scarred by the time they even realized they had an infection. Their male partners were rarely diagnosed or treated. Medical experts said that almost half of the raging infections caused by pelvic inflammatory disease (PID) went untreated until they had seriously scarred or destroyed a woman's fallopian tubes. The most common of the infections, chlamydia, caused about four million new cases every year. Federal health officials said the increase in gonorrhea and chlamydia was largely to blame for record levels of ectopic pregnancies. The life-threatening complication, in which the fetus developed outside the womb, had nearly quadrupled in the past 20 years, affecting almost 17 out of every 1,000 pregnancies. In 1987, the most recent year for which figures were available, 88,000 women were hospitalized with ectopic pregnancies, an increase of 19 percent over the previous year. The condition not only cost the woman her pregnancy, but it often left her fallopian tubes and ovaries so scarred that the only way she could conceive again was with the help of an infertility clinic.

The diseases were "nearly out of control," medical authorities said. Yet, allowing for inflation, the government spent less in 1989 on controlling sexually transmitted diseases than it did in 1943. The victims of such diseases were members of what Dr. Willard Cates of the U.S. Centers for Disease Control would call "a politically disenfranchised, voiceless population."

Yet it was hard to think of the well-dressed white couples in the Norfolk waiting room as disenfranchised in any conventional sense. "A good percentage of our patients are lawyers and doctors," said clinic coordinator Catherine H. Kruithoff. "They certainly are well-educated, upper middle class for the most part. A good portion are second marriages. Less than fifteen percent of the patients have substantial insurance coverage for this. So for most of them it is all out of pocket." Black couples were half again as likely to be infertile as white couples. So were couples in which the wife had not finished high school. The poor were hardest hit. But they were not in evidence in waiting rooms at Norfolk and other infertility clinics.

In the library, a nurse met with the new patients to outline the different experiments open to them. Reproductive health studies. Ovulation drug trials. Doppler ultrasound studies. Endometrial biopsies. They thumbed through consent forms. A new embryo-freezing protocol. No charge for that one; there wasn't any pregnancy rate established yet. "If you want to maximize your opportunities while you are here, this may be the study for you," said Linda Wilkins, another clinic coordinator. The couples took notes. "The next person you need to see is our bookkeeper," she said.

The sun was setting. The women were leaving as quickly as they arrived. They would be back in the early morning, some for shots, some for egg collection, some to receive their embryos. A few would be canceled. One woman in a black sweat shirt and blue jeans lingered to talk. She was a lawyer. She, too, was nearing forty. She already had one child through IVF; now she was trying for a second. Her hip was sore from an injection of Pergonal. She slouched sideways in her seat so she wouldn't sit directly on the needle puncture.

Most of what she knew about infertility, she said, she learned as an attorney defending the Dalkon Shield in one of thousands of lawsuits filed against it. No, she had never worn one. Her fallopian tubes were blocked. The egg produced every month in her ovaries had no way to reach her uterus; that door to her womb was locked. She didn't know why.

"You come back to the clinic because it's the only thing that you can do, the only hope that you have to have a baby," she said. "Instead of just feeling very sad and despairing, you make an appointment to come back one more time because then you are doing something."

Risa York stood under the awning outside the surgical and diagnostic unit at Sentara Norfolk General Hospital, waiting nervously for her husband, Steven, to emerge. It was 11:21 A.M. on September 25, 1989. She was not allowed to enter the clinic where she had been a patient.

An expert in reproductive law from the American Bar Foundation, a local attorney, three television crews, and eight reporters waited with her. After a 28-month battle in federal district court, the Jones Clinic had given up possession of the couple's only frozen embryo. Steven York had gone inside to claim it.

In all, the couple had conceived 12 embryos in the Norfolk laboratory. Eleven were used in three unsuccessful attempts to get Risa York pregnant. The twelfth was frozen for safekeeping. When the Yorks sought to transfer it from Norfolk to an equally reputable clinic in Los Angeles, the Jones Institute balked. A simple contest of wills between doctor and patient edged into unexplored legal territory.

The dispute set two people who were not yet parents against doctors who were not quite legal guardians over custody of something that was not yet a child and not exactly a patient. The clinic said it was guided "by its perception of the highest standard of medical practice and ethics, as well as the establishment of the best public policy in this area." Many of their colleagues, however, disagreed sharply. The Yorks had no reason to feel intimidated by a doctor's judgment. Steven York was a successful Los Angeles physician, himself well schooled in medical ethics.

"We feel physicians have no right to exert dominion over a couple's genetic material," Risa York said. "The embryo is potentially our child."

When Steven York emerged from the hospital, he carried in his right hand a humble victory trophy—a steel-gray thermos secured with a red cap. Their embryo was inside, frozen at 186 degrees Celsius in a glass straw resembling a cocktail swizzle stick. Howard and Georgeanna Jones followed a few steps behind. In their green surgical scrubs and masks, the two elderly infertility experts looked like something from a Norman Rockwell painting—the living portrait of medical rectitude. Howard Jones, the grandfather of laboratory conception, fielded questions in a voice as deep and melodious as a concert bassoon. Georgeanna Jones smiled with her lips parted, her eyebrows raised in an air of pleased expectation. In front of the photographers, the smile would freeze and the eyes would flash with impatient intelligence. She did not suffer fools.

In the national debate over the beginning of life, the Yorks's embryo set a minor precedent. U.S. District Judge Calvitt Clarke, Jr., ruled that the embryo was property. Six days earlier, a Tennessee state judge had ruled that a frozen embryo was a frozen human being. Doctors called it a zygote, a pre-zygote, a pre-embryo, or a fertilized egg. Whatever it was, the two-year-old cluster of cells sat on the seat next to Risa York on American Airlines Flight 75 bound for Los Angeles. Was it a passenger or an extra piece of carry-on luggage? The Yorks took no chances; they bought it a ticket. By 2:30 P.M., it was airborne.

It would be left for legal analysts to sort out the conflicting rulings. One aspect of the case was unambiguous. The Jones clinic had exercised its medical authority and been publicly rebuffed—first by its patients, then by a federal judge. The clinic agreed to pay $17,500 to cover the Yorks's legal expenses. In their long career, the Joneses had faced down anti-abortion demonstrators, outfoxed hostile politicians, and built a $50 million research institute from scratch. Now, perhaps for the first time, they had been overruled as the medical court of last resort.

The clinic would have to get used to patients who thought for themselves. The doctors added more patient meetings, scheduled a lecture series, and offered afternoon teas. They quietly inserted a new clause in the patient consent forms. From now on, any human embryos frozen in Norfolk would have to be thawed there, as well.

What infertile couples called an illness, earlier generations had been content to call fate.

If couples felt exploited and powerless in their private distress, they fought like the Yorks for public control. They were some of the most assertive and articulate members of their generation. Where some had once mobilized for the Equal Rights Amendment, others had formed the front ranks of the Reagan revolution. They all came of age in an era when government was expected to ensure the public health: to inspect routinely the meat they ate, to fluoridate the water they drank, and to monitor the dye in the cherries on their ice-cream sundaes. But in their struggle to conceive, many couples felt abandoned.

So they organized. They litigated. They picketed. They built a national support group. They set up hotlines and published newsletters. They aired their anguish on television talk shows and in countless newspaper articles. They turned family itself into a political issue. They spurred congressional hearings in 1988 and again in 1989. With an eye to attracting more media coverage, they arranged for celebrities to testify.

Their aggression was a response to abuse. Too many couples had been burned by indifferent or inexpert infertility specialists. Doctors rarely told their patients when success rates dropped or if key laboratory personnel changed. The field was so rife with fraud and misleading claims that the American Fertility Society felt obliged to issue a formal statement on advertising standards.

The case of Vicki Earhardt and her husband, Bill, was every couple's cautionary nightmare. For a decade, the Virginia couple tried to conceive a child, spending $35,000 on fertility drugs and high-tech reproductive methods—all to no avail. Seven times her doctor told her she was pregnant. Seven times her doctor told her her body had "absorbed" the fetus. When congressional investigators subsequently reviewed her medical records, they confirmed what she had come to suspect—she had never been pregnant at all. "Each time I felt like I had failed again, that my own body was killing our baby. But then I would get that urge again and want a baby so badly that I would go through anything," she testified in 1988.

Infertile couples often found themselves doing the medical homework their doctors neglected. They became educated consumers who talked knowingly of "embryo management." Time made many infertile couples coldly pragmatic. When they needed money to underwrite their organizing efforts, they did more than hold fund-raising dinners or weekend car washes. The couples who had sued A. H. Robins, Searle, Squibb, Eli Lilly, Abbott, and other medical conglomerates over the products that caused their infertility allied themselves with other major pharmaceutical firms that sold fertility drugs. The hormones they manufactured caused severe mood swings, cysts, and the risk of long-term side effects. Because the hormones themselves were toxic at high levels, they interfered with the embryo's ability to implant. University of California researchers linked one of the most popularly prescribed fertility drugs to birth defects. The researchers found that clomophene citrate, which could linger for weeks after a woman stopped taking it, could cause defects in the reproductive system of a fetus not unlike those caused by the drug DES.

From companies like Sandoz Pharmaceuticals Corp. and Serono Laboratories Inc. came the money for patient-education seminars and glossy pamphlets on infertility. When Resolve, a national infertility support group, celebrated its fifteenth anniversary with a gala three-day conference in Washington, D.C., Ares-Serono sponsored the event. When Resolve issued a press release, printed on handsome pink stock, to alert the media to "the children that science made possible," the fine print at the bottom would note that the cost was covered by Sandoz Pharmaceuticals. The press release extolled the virtues of the company's newest fertility drug. In fine print, a product data sheet would report that the drug was linked to alarming changes in blood pressure, strokes, seizures, and a handful of heart attacks. The company noted that the relationship between the adverse side effects and the drug "is not certain."

Putting infertile couples together with the drug companies was a marketing marriage made in heaven. "It's a win-win situation," said one Serono executive. "We help people learn more about infertility treatment and we increase our market share."

Serono Laboratories President Thomas G. Wiggans said his company's formula for success was straightforward: "An educated patient is a loyal patient. An educated patient is more likely to either seek therapy, seek continued therapy, talk to his or her friends about seeking therapy. I wouldn't sit here and tell you there aren't market development components to this educational approach, because clearly there are. It's a symbiotic relationship."

One of Serono's many pamphlets urged couples to pressure employers to cover the costs of infertility treatments like those the company sold. The company gave Resolve $40,000 to lobby through its 50 local chapters for changes in state insurance laws across the country so that employers would pay for infertility treatments. Working through Resolve, the company lobbied heavily for new insurance laws in Massachusetts and California. When Resolve proposed an insurance reform handbook, detailing how to lobby a state legislature, Serono paid for the printing and made sure copies went to every Resolve chapter in the country.

By 1990, after less than five years, legislation was pending in 20 states requiring insurance companies to pay for the infertility procedures. Five legislatures had already passed laws. If you were a politician, it was always hard to argue against motherhood. "We sent Baby Jesus Christmas cards to all the legislators," one volunteer lobbyist in Wisconsin recalled with satisfaction. "We sent it to their home address so their wives would think about it."

It was raining outside that September afternoon, but inside New York Hospital, Sev Rosenwaks was having a sunny day.

The staff knew the signs. His whistle preceded him through the corridors. Walking briskly with his hands clasped behind him, he cut a striking figure: broad shoulders in a pressed white lab coat, broad cheekbones, heavy-lidded blue eyes, and a wave of blond hair over his forehead. He held his head cocked at a jaunty angle. He exuded a self-assurance and tranquility that bordered on arrogance.

Rosenwaks was beaming. It had been barely a year since he had resigned from Norfolk, but he felt ahead of even his own ambitious schedule. The clinic's operating budget had grown to about $5 million a year. Its pregnancy rate had stabilized at an enviable level. He had started a donor egg program. He was preparing the foundation for embryo surgery. Within a year, he wanted to offer high-risk patients the ability to perform prenatal diagnosis on their embryos. His blueprints for expansion were ready; he wanted to double the clinic's size and staff right off the bat. And he had just hired Jacques Cohen.

The money was in place. Dr. William Ledger, the hospital's chief of obstetrics and gynecology, held the check aloft like a laurel wreath. The mother of a grateful patient had given them $500,000. It was worth that much to her to become a grandmother. He showed it to every nurse in the hall. "All the happiness in the world can't buy you money," Ledger said. Within days, the donor would double it. Within weeks, the construction crews started tearing out the walls.

When Rosenwaks moved to Manhattan in 1988, *New York Magazine* heralded the arrival of a "new fertility god." *Manhattan Inc.*, with an eye to the clinic's financial statement, called him New York Hospital's baby-maker, money-maker, and image-maker. So far he had lived up to his promise.

As Rosenwaks outlined his plans, his voice resonated with the echo of his Israeli birthplace. When he was twelve years old, his family moved to Flatbush, Brooklyn. He won a medical school fellowship at Johns Hopkins University, where he impressed two professors in particular: Howard and Georgeanna Jones. When the Joneses organized the institute that would bear their name, they thought of their young protégé and invited him to become its first medical director. By that time, his former professors had already made 30 babies in the laboratory. Rosenwaks had never practiced IVF, but by the time he left, he was a world authority who had helped create 450 babies.

By leaving Norfolk, he took a giant step out from under the shadow of Howard and Georgeanna Jones. Even if he had helped write the definitive text on laboratory conception at Norfolk, his was the last in the list of authors' names on its cover. Whatever new program Rosenwaks could build at Cornell—in one of the country's biggest and best-known hospitals—would be a measure of his own stature. As Cornell's new infertility guru, his profile couldn't be higher. If he could not match the sheer size of the Jones Institute, he could make up for it in energy and ambition.

"Norfolk was becoming a self-perpetuating entity that had little to do with the personalities in it," he explained. "I wanted to do my own thing and pursue the areas I thought were important. I think Norfolk, because it was first and is an excellent clinic, was getting to the point where basically it was doing the same thing over and over again. Not as much innovation. I have a peculiar personality in medicine; I like new concepts. Someone else can work out all the details."

Rosenwaks believed that the field badly needed innovation. For more than five years, doctors tinkered with the same techniques, constantly refining them with almost no improvement in overall success rates. His former colleagues at Norfolk didn't disagree. They believed it was the nature of the field itself, however, not the Jones Institute. "We are at a plateau now," said Dr. Anibal Acosta, the surgeon on the team that produced the first U.S. test-tube baby. "For a while, we made major leaps in IVF. We ran. We skipped ahead. Now to make any progress, we must crawl."

Rosenwaks was in no mood to crawl. Laboratory conception had opened a window into the entire human reproduction system. He wanted to explore the world it revealed. "You're looking at how things fundamentally work," he said. "You have to be willing to try new things."

More than his own ambition was at work. The reputation of New York Hospital—with 1,462 beds, 2,931 doctors, and

2,001 nurses—was tarnished by allegations of medical mishaps and accidental deaths. A world-class IVF clinic could rehabilitate that reputation. At least hospital administrators hoped so.

Outside the hospital, other pressures were building. At congressional hearings during 1988 and 1989, witnesses called low IVF success rates a national disgrace. In 1989, the Federal Trade Commission opened an investigation into advertising practices among IVF clinics. The U.S. General Accounting Office also started questioning human embryo laboratories. The American Fertility Society was writing its first laboratory standards. Congress was framing legislation to bring the industry to heel. In Washington, as the Reagan administration relinquished power and the Bush administration assumed it, rumors were spreading that for the first time in almost 20 years the federal government might authorize funding for research on human reproduction.

In Atlanta, Jacques Cohen was intrigued. He wanted more time and resources for his embryo research. In Holland and England, his work had been blocked by clinical caution and politics. He bubbled with ideas, but he could never try them out as quickly as he wanted to.

"I need a physician who is very keen," said Cohen, as he considered Rosenwaks and the move to New York. "I am dependent on a clinician who is keen. He may be the one. He is very keen indeed."

It was rush hour in the Cornell laboratory. Mina Alikani sat on the edge of her seat to position her eyes properly at the microscope, her back arched, her elbows out, almost like a virtuoso addressing a grand piano. She had barely moved since early morning.

"You know, when we asked that man to produce a second sperm sample, he really got quite angry. He said: At my age, you must be kidding." She would thaw some from his stock of frozen sperm, then use it to fortify his specimen.

She would spin the sperm in a centrifuge, then allow it to sit until the strongest sperm had kicked to the top of the tube. Those she would skim off and then repeat the procedure, until she had collected a concentrated sample of the healthiest cells he had produced. Only those would be used to fertilize his wife's eggs. With her centrifuge and test tubes, Mina Alikani had supplanted natural selection. Inside the lab, she was an evolutionary force under whose care only the very fittest would be allowed to reproduce.

For the moment, Alikani kept her eyes pasted to the microscope. She had to judge the maturity of each human egg to gauge the best time for fertilization. There were eight so far from this patient and they were bloody. Every one got a grade.

"I don't think any of these will be fertilized before midnight. That makes the life of an embryologist less than desirable," said Alikani. She used two glass dissecting needles to free the egg before the blood clot could poison it. The needle in her left hand pinned the egg down, while the right needle picked away the debris.

McVicker passed her the next tube. She poured it into a petri dish, scanned it, and dumped it. Nothing. Her hands blurred. Five more dishes ended up in the waste bag.

"This woman has been through this several times," Alikani said. "She is very young, very beautiful. Unfortunately, her body does not like to get pregnant. Her hormonal picture is questionable. She gets wonderful embryos, but she doesn't get pregnant."

Alikani had been in New York seven months and had barely stepped outside the lab. A wiry Australian embryologist named Ian Pike taught her the craft in California. By only a small coincidence, Pike's Australian colleagues had organized the original Cornell embryo laboratory. The world of human egg pushers and embryo jockeys was so small that they could all waltz comfortably in one medium-sized hotel ballroom. The Australians were its dance masters, teaching the new technology's latest two-step in every country. Pike taught Alikani. Alikani taught McVicker. Jacques Cohen's system differed so radically from Cornell's that, when he took over the laboratory later in 1989, Alikani would apprentice again. The field changed so quickly that there was no time to write the textbooks or organize the university courses. She would have to watch over his shoulder.

"One more tube," said McVicker.

"Now we're done?" asked Alikani.

"Now we're done."

They reviewed the last patient's tote sheet. Twelve eggs in all, each catalogued on a clinical report card. They sorted the worst into one batch.

McVicker held up the dish. "Are these all her question marks?"

In all, the doctors collected 72 eggs from a half-dozen women that September morning. For the embryologists, that meant 72 eggs to grade, to fertilize later that evening; 72 eggs to inspect for signs of fertilization the following day. Each egg took 75 seconds to inspect. While those embryos matured in the incubators, dozens more eggs would be collected and fertilized every day. There would be dozens more to check, to culture and transfer or freeze. At the end of the week, they would have at least that many embryos to replace. It went on like that every day without respite for 30 to 40 days at a stretch.

"What can we do? This is Egg Central," said Alikani. She checked the digital thermometers on the four embryo incubators. Each was set at body temperature. The incubators were, in their fashion, also waiting rooms.

While the men and women waited for their turn with the embryologists, they were haunted by their expectations and their sense of failure.

Kathy Hecht,* a diminutive bookkeeper, had a recurring dream. As she sat with her husband in traffic on Boston's Southeast Expressway, inching toward their morning appointment at a hospital infertility clinic, she wondered again if she should tell him about it. It was always the same dream, and every morning she found a reason to keep it to herself.

They were native New Englanders, Jewish, the first in their college crowd to marry, and the last still trying, unsuccessfully, to conceive their first child. She wanted to adopt a child, just as her parents had adopted her. But adoption agency bureaucracies had consumed years of her time without producing anything more than a waiting list. Now she was thirty-nine years old. Several of her friends had had children with the help of infertility specialists, but this was her first attempt. It didn't matter to her whether she actually had a baby of her own, she said; it mattered that she tried.

So she sat in traffic, remembering her dream: The doctors had made an embryo for her. It divided into two halves that fit neatly in her hands. In her right hand, they placed a perfectly formed miniature human being. In her left, they placed an undifferentiated mass of cells, like a blob from a jellyfish washed up on the beach. Those cells were useless, the doctors would tell her; discard them. But keep the little human, they said. They would use that later. They sealed the embryo in a bell jar and entrusted it to her for safekeeping. In the dream, when the day came to implant the embryo inside her, she brought the container back to the laboratory. When the doctors opened it, they only found the formless mass of cells inside. We can't use this, they told her. Didn't we give you the one that was good?

"And I had lost it. Then I wake up. Somewhere inside of me I feel like I'm totally responsible. I don't feel that when I'm awake, but inside me there's something saying it's all my fault," she said. "This is what my body is supposed to be capable of doing. I think, please let me be able to do this just one time, because people are watching. My most private and uncontrolled behavior is being observed by a lot of people. I just hope that I ovulate, that the egg is normal, and that they can retrieve it."

Kathy wondered again if she should tell her husband the dream.

3

Lisa Fagg's Thanksgiving

She rocked slowly in the sun-room, watching the warm patch of light crawl across the carpet. There was a basket of fresh daisies, carnations, and cattails on the table. Porcelain birds roosted on a sideboard. A dog barked in the bedroom. She sipped lemonade. She felt herself oddly off balance, her attention centered completely on two swelling specks of tissue deep inside her body.

On Thanksgiving Day, 1989, an embryologist at Reproductive Biology Associates operated on two embryos and then transferred them to her womb. The embryos had been altered in an experiment designed by Jacques Cohen.

Today, she was not yet pregnant. She was not unpregnant, either. In her rocking chair, she was suspended between the two states in a precarious new condition for which there was not yet an etiquette or a proper vocabulary. In this unclaimed territory, she was only an observer. In her uterus, the two embryos actively struggled to secure their beachhead on existence. She was, for the moment, an introspective container.

It would be 12 days before the most sensitive clinical tests could detect a pregnancy. Only then would she know whether the embryos had implanted in her uterus, whether they would collaborate with her in a pregnancy. In the interim, she balanced anticipation and elation, exhaustion and dread. She rocked.

Lisa Fagg, aged thirty, did her best to be comfortable. She lounged in a red-and-lavender track suit. The radio played softly in the background. But she was attuned to a reproductive transformation that most women underwent unknowingly. Some were more sensitive to their bodies than others; some women taught themselves to recognize the twinge of muscle at the precise moment they ovulated. But this was something more subtle. This preceded even the most intuitive knowledge of pregnancy.

Prior to implantation, the embryo is naturally hidden within the body's shell. An egg emerges from the ovary, coaxed by the feathery edges of the fallopian tube brushing the curve of the ovary like a graceful anemone. The egg enters the fallopian tube, where it encounters a single sperm. The two cells fuse to become one, floating in the water of life—a fluid with the same salt content as the sea. For conception to occur properly, the egg must join the sperm before its first day outside the ovary is finished. As it moves toward the entrance to the uterus, the newly fertilized egg rides on a continuous wave stirred by beds of microscopic cilia that line the fallopian tube. The journey may take up to four days. By the time it reaches the uterus, the single transformed cell has become a tightly packed sphere of more than 100 cells. Still, there is no chemical hint of its presence. For days, the embryo then floats freely into the uterus, where, perhaps, it will implant and, in its first public manifestation, trigger the overt physical signals of pregnancy.

The act of implantation transforms the embryo and the woman who carries it. When it arrives in the uterus, the embryo still has not settled on its own identity. It has the potential to become one person, or a crowd. Its cells could yield twins, triplets, or quadruplets. Implantation is a moment of biological commitment. The embryo's outer layer of cells penetrates the wall of the uterus to become the placenta. The remaining inner cell mass becomes the mature embryo. What transforms the embryo also changes the woman that carries it. It alters her body chemistry and her knowledge of herself. She becomes an expectant mother.

Most embryos never implant. They may stick in the folds and twists of the fallopian tube. They may jam in the constricted opening to the uterus. They may bounce for days against the soft walls and ceiling of uterine tissue, unable to burst free of the transparent zona sheath and implant. Whatever the cause, their demise is neither noted nor mourned. Only one in four actually develops into a living child.

That natural journey—traversing a distance of less than five inches—is a fundamental voyage made by a free-living, biologically independent entity, the primordial precursor of the passage every human makes into the breathing world. Technology made that microscopic journey into a medical procedure. In vitro fertilization laid it bare in a plastic dish and made plain its essential independence, so that, even when it vanished again into the womb, its afterimage lingered.

As she rocked, Lisa Fagg wondered if these embryos would survive inside her. She could still feel the swelling and soreness inside her from the doctor's needle. Her system was still woozy from the drugs she had taken to stimulate the production of multiple eggs. "You get so many injections," she said. "Some days, I was getting four injections a day." Her ovaries were so swollen she felt as if someone had kicked her in the stomach. It was a symptom of a potentially fatal side effect called hyperstimulation. If the doses of hormones were too strong, the ovaries could literally explode.

In the laboratory, she had seen on a video screen the two embryos now within her. On her bedroom dresser, she placed a photograph of them both taken in the minute before they were placed inside her. They looked like soap bubbles.

For the next two weeks, it would be the last thing she and her husband, Bill, would look at every evening, the first thing every morning—"for luck," they said. They could, if they wished, give them names. They could, if they wished, know their sex and their susceptibility to inherited diseases. If they wanted, they could have had their embryos carried to term by another woman. They could, if any embryologist dared, have the two cloned into four, eight, or 16 identical duplicates. It was the fourth time in a year she had arrived at this point. Three times before the embryos failed to implant. Ten embryos had died inside her.

She kept photographs of them all, pressed between the brown-leather covers of her wedding album like bridal flowers. There was the Polaroid of the three from November 1988; the three from the following May; the four from August. "I teased my husband that the one in the middle looked just like him," she said.

Five more embryos conceived in August had been frozen to be used another day. The photographs, the embryos, and the cells in storage had cost them more than the $28,000 the doctors had charged.

"We've lost ten children that are in heaven," she said. "We look to the future and the five frozen that are left to be born. We have two babies that are hopefully still alive right now inside me, but this time next week they may not be. It's something you want so badly and so desperately and you have no control over it and it really hurts."

When Lisa and Bill arose that Thanksgiving Day, they were elated by the sheer number of eggs they had incubating in the laboratory. Doctors had siphoned 13 eggs from her ovaries. The couple expected most of them to fertilize. Because the clinic would transfer no more than three embryos to her womb at any one time, to reduce the risk of triplets and quadruplets, the surplus embryos could be frozen and added to their "stash" of stored embryos.

This embryo supply was a matter of money and, for Lisa Fagg, the growing realization that she could not face another full round of hormone shots, egg retrievals, and transfers.

In addition, their insurance also would soon be exhausted. If they were to continue in their pursuit of a biological child, they must turn to a cheaper and less-disruptive method. They calculated the cost of replacing a frozen embryo at about one-sixth that of a full in vitro fertilization cycle, in which doctors would have to stimulate and retrieve fresh eggs. Each new frozen embryo was worth its weight, if not in gold, then in hope.

"I wanted to add more to my stash," Bill said. "Was I getting greedy? I don't look at it as being greedy. I look at it as having more opportunities."

Instead, for reasons neither they nor the doctors would ever adequately explain, only two eggs quickened into embryos. Lying on the examination table, ready to receive the two embryos, Lisa felt the old sense of desperation well inside her. With so few embryos to transfer and none to save for another attempt later, the odds she would become pregnant abruptly turned against her. But there would be no public displays of disappointment for either of them. Her husband kissed her on the forehead.

"I looked at Lisa and I knew she wanted to cry, and I wanted to cry, but we wanted to be happy because we had two. I wanted to cry all day yesterday and I just couldn't," Bill said.

It was Thanksgiving Day. Relatives were in the living room. There was a family dinner to serve, appearances to keep up. She was not allowed to move for 24 hours after the embryo transfer. Her husband set the formal table and cooked the turkey. He cleared the tableware, washed the dishes, and, at dusk, walked the dogs. He was a big man with a stern, sad, handsome face, a homespun mountain Presbyterian from North Carolina. He came across as a plainspoken man who did his duty stoically, no matter how great the personal inconvenience, like a pine mast just supple enough to give in a gale. Now he found himself in a storm of emotions. He was having a hard time finding the strength to bend.

"You're mad at God and you're mad at the world. You do try to stay on an even keel. I basically hold it in. It's probably taking its toll inside me because I do hold it in," he said. "That night, I wanted to cry so bad. I just wanted to go outside and cry because I was hurting so bad. But I had to fix the dinner. I had to eat the dinner, clean up. I took the dogs for a walk. I went outside and I wanted to cry, but I couldn't. I still held it in. I've got a bad taste in my mouth right now."

Lisa rocked in her chair. Two embryos floated on the fluids of her womb. Her husband walked in the dark.

It was a step they had vowed they would never take, then promised they would never repeat, and finally found almost impossible to resist. It became something for which Lisa was willing to reject her Church and her parents' Catholic faith. "They'll baptize the children. They may excommunicate me, but they will welcome the children," she said.

It transformed a shy woman into a community activist who buttonholed state legislators about adoption and insurance reform bills as persistently as the boldest professional lobbyist. She overcame her qualms and volunteered as a human research subject. Lisa and Bill Fagg made themselves medical statistics. Theirs was a clinical trial.

"We are experiments," she said.

They met in Mobile, Alabama. He was the branch manager of a furniture-leasing company, and she was a leasing agent. She was nineteen; he was twenty-nine. He liked her curly hair, her garnet eyes, and freckles. On their first date, they dined at Russo's in Mobile. He was celebrating his thirtieth birthday. Several tables away, a large family dined. "I just kept my eyes on the kids. One or two of them came up to me and I played with them. Lisa knew we would have to have lots of kids if we ever got married," he said.

"Bill said he wanted a whole household full," she recalled.

He proposed on the night before Thanksgiving 1979. They picked out the ring together and married the following May. They never used birth control. But she didn't become pregnant until three years later—an ectopic pregnancy that ruptured before it was diagnosed.

"I was on the floor sick, doubled over in pain. I remember thinking, 'God, if this is what it means to be pregnant, I don't know if I want it or not,' " Lisa said. Three times, her husband drove her to the emergency room. Three times the doctors sent her away. The fourth time, she was rushed into surgery. They changed doctors.

More important for them, they started to attend meetings of the support group Resolve. They sat quietly in the back rows during meetings and "soaked it up like sponges," Lisa said. They couldn't read the pamphlets and books fast enough. She volunteered to take calls on the chapter's hotline. She discovered she was a natural community organizer. Within months, she became chapter president. The hours once given to uncertainty over their ability to start a family were now filled with the business of setting up symposia and chapter meetings. The doctors quickly learned to recognize her name on the schedule of patients. "Ah, yes," Dr. Massey at RBA said dryly, "the Queen of Resolve." Bill and Lisa also added their name to the adoption list at Catholic Social Services. Adoption would cost about $9,000. The agency placed only about 15 babies a year, and its waiting list was measured in years.

Three times surgeons operated on her fallopian tubes. One was scarred beyond repair, the other badly damaged. Such operations could cause as many problems as they were meant to solve. Pelvic surgery often left new adhesions and scars that made it even harder for a woman to conceive.

In their new world sex was scheduled like car maintenance. No one called it sex; it became "assisted reproductive technology." Couples didn't fail; they had a "response." The doctors used language as a refuge from the rage and grief that confronted them in their offices every day. It kept them balanced high on the medical pedestal. Doctors spoke dryly of "fecundability patterns" and "adequate abstinence intervals" and "artifactually elevated sperm counts." When the couples discussed their own bodies, they adopted the jargon. They sounded like NASA engineers explaining away the latest space shuttle launch delay. Bill and Lisa dug in their heels.

"When we first talked about it, we said there was no way we would go through in vitro," she said. "We were concerned the children would not be normal." On her own, she sought out children conceived in the laboratory so she could assure herself they were not freaks. "I wanted to see that these kids were healthy and normal and cried the same way as other children."

Their third infertility specialist referred them to Hilton Kort, at Reproductive Biology Associates. They waited almost six months for an appointment. By the time they got in to see him, they had been on the adoption waiting list three and a half years. Lisa turned thirty; Bill turned forty.

They were willing to risk the technology, but they promised themselves they would go through this only once. They knew the odds of success were remote. They assured themselves that they would be the one-in-ten couple—the couple for whom it worked perfectly the first time.

"We were very adamant about that. We'd do it once and that's it," Lisa said. "I think within a week after the first negative pregnancy test, we were on the phone to schedule a consultation with the doctor to get in on the next IVF cycle."

Failure made them bold. Each time they tried again, they volunteered for a new experiment, in the hopes that it would improve their chances. They allowed their embryos to be frozen. They agreed to take new hormones. The clinic prescribed steroids and, although she was mildly allergic, Lisa took those, too. They agreed to let Jacques Cohen perform microsurgery on her unfertilized eggs, then on the embryos themselves. They allowed Cohen to attempt the genetic repair of their defective embryos. They signed up for Cohen's "hatching" experiment. She consented to carry the altered embryos in her womb.

The couple who had begun so opposed to the technology stepped into its vanguard. However, the new procedures couldn't relieve the emotional distress. Lisa turned down a raise and a promotion because she would have to move away from the clinic. Then she quit her job. Relatives wondered aloud about the emotional strain. A close friend volunteered to become their surrogate mother. When another infertile friend announced that she had chosen "child-free" living, Lisa didn't know what to say. They lied to their friends about how many times they had tried and failed in the laboratory. At night, she would tearfully tell Bill to divorce her for someone who could bear his children.

On their third attempt, they agreed to try a new drug called Lupron—the trade name for a synthetic hormone called leuprolide acetate, manufactured by Japan's largest pharmaceutical company, Takeda Chemical Industries, in partnership with Abbott Laboratories. Lupron was so powerful it could shut down the woman's entire hormonal system in a temporary menopause. The drug was becoming increasingly popular among infertility specialists because it effectively allowed them to turn a woman's hormonal system on and off like a faucet.

There had never been a systematic study of its long-term effects on women or on a pregnancy. The U.S. Food and Drug Administration had only approved it as a chemotherapy agent for men with prostate cancer. Like the natural gonadotropin-releasing hormone it imitates, leuprolide regulates menstrual cycles and the release of the male sex hormone by signaling the pituitary gland to secrete follicle-stimulating hormone and luteinizing hormone in both men and women. Those hormones, in turn, control the production of sperm and eggs. In 1989, Takeda took in $63 million from U.S. sales of Lupron. No one could tell how much of it had been sold as a cancer remedy or as an infertility treatment. It was so powerful an inhibitor of the body's hormones that doctors could use it to delay the onset of sexual maturity for years in children suffering from central precocious puberty, a rare disorder that triggered sexual maturity in children.

"It was kind of scary," Lisa Fagg said. "We felt we were really playing with my body here." They were unknowingly playing with their embryos, as well. Scientists like Cohen noticed that Lupron embryos were different. They grew faster, developed more rapidly. They were more fragile when frozen and less likely to survive thawing. Nobody knew why or what it meant for the long-term health of the woman or any resulting child.

"We don't know what all this is doing to her body, all these drugs, steroids, all the multiple eggs, everything," her husband said. "I have no idea what it's going to do to her body in the long term and how it will affect her."

They pored over the consent forms together for hours. "I think you have to know to ask the right questions," she said. "You can sign your life away on those little forms and not really know what you're signing." She listened intently as Massey and Kort outlined the experiments at Resolve meetings. They both knew Catholic doctrine on in vitro fertilization. "Through these procedures, with apparently contrary purposes, life and death are subjected to the decision of man, who thus sets himself up as the giver of life and death by decree. This dynamic of violence and domination may remain unnoticed by those very individuals who, wishing to utilize this procedure, become subject to it themselves." They sought advice from Catholic friends, but they were not willing to discuss it with a priest.

Bill signed with few illusions. "I am a guinea pig. We are guinea pigs. There were guinea pigs before us," he said. "This is our only alternative to get Lisa pregnant. We've had to do what we've had to do. We had to put our faith in their hands, and we did."

The hatch window snapped open in the darkened operating room. A pair of eyes appeared. It was Jacques Cohen. Violins and cellos could be heard behind him. The nurse handed him a single tube of strawberry-colored fluid. His face withdrew. In a moment, his voice drifted out with the music: "Egg. And another one."

On the operating table, Lisa Fagg drifted on the edge of consciousness. She was wired into machines. It seemed easier this time, she thought. What was this, the third? It was August 12, 1989. Dr. Hilton Kort, with an ultrasound probe and aspiration needle, searched her ovaries for egg follicles. He turned the probe one way and then the other. On the video monitor to his left, the ultrasound scan painted her interior landscape. Each follicle containing an egg appeared as a black sphere.

Kort guided the needle in, punctured the sphere, and then, operating a suction pump, drained its contents. Kort steered the needle by watching the screen. It required the same kind of disconnected hand and eye coordination as a complicated video game. The fluid was siphoned through a connecting hose into a test tube. The nurse passed each new tube through the hatch.

Cohen's voice returned: "Egg. Another one. Egg."

Kort shifted the probe. "Lisa, you are going to feel a little stick."

She groaned.

The nature of the procedure lent a disembodied quality to the scene. Nobody watched the patient directly; she was overshadowed by her own ultrasound image. It formed a bright video window into her womb. The small open hatch into the embryo laboratory, like the monitor, also was an opening into that remote, interior world. Unseen from the operating room, Cohen and the embryologists manipulated cells that normally belonged inside her ovaries and her uterus. For a moment, it seemed as if the lab itself was actually inside her.

Jacques Cohen diced the smear of cells surrounding the egg under the microscope. There was so much blood in the ovarian fluid that he had trouble spotting her eggs even under intense magnification. Twenty minutes after the operating room had cleared, Cohen was still panning for eggs. By the time he discarded the last tube, he had found 11. His eyes were pink with strain.

For the next two days, the eggs were his. They would live in his laboratory incubators. Nine would become embryos. Some would become candidates for surgery. Others he would seal in glass ampules with a blowtorch and freeze in liquid nitrogen. The eggs and embryos were like snowflakes—no two quite alike, physically or genetically. The cells around them swirled in fanciful shapes like clouds on a summer's day. Cumulus cells, the embryologists had named them.

Cohen worked in relative darkness, prospecting by the greenish light from the lamp underneath the microscope stage. He worked in the dark, he said, because human eggs and embryos naturally were never exposed to daylight, and excessive exposure to certain wavelengths of light could damage them. Cohen cleaned each egg and moved it into a drop of culture medium. The drop was itself encapsulated in mineral oil, effectively sealing it from the outside world. Floating in the oil, the embryo inside the droplet was shielded from lethal changes in acidity, abrupt temperature shifts, dust, and the natural exchange of gases in the air. If allowed to reach room temperature for even 10 minutes, a human egg could develop chromosomal abnormalities.

He sorted the 11 eggs into their droplets under the microscope, etched the mother and father's name on the underside of the dish that held the eggs, and slid it into the incubator. The term "test-tube baby" had become a permanent part of the English language, but in most labs the test tubes themselves had long since become obsolete. Cohen's assistant, embryologist Graham Wright, had used them in England. They figured prominently in his nightmares.

"You'd have a rack for each patient with a bunch of these tubes. Each tube had one egg or one embryo. Every time you wanted to look at one, you had to put a poker in, find the embryo, and pull it out of the tube," Wright said. Every inspection increased the risk of damaging the embryo. In the same laboratory, they found that the fastest way to deliver sperm samples from the fifth-floor clinic to the basement laboratory was to drop them in a padded envelope off the fire escape. "You'd hear a thud in the courtyard," Wright recalled. "Sometimes the wind would blow one onto the roof of the garage next door." They painted crosshairs on the courtyard to improve their accuracy.

Cohen spared his eggs and embryos any rough handling. An embryologist could inspect them through the optically transparent oil without ever disturbing them. For his purposes, the oil technique had an even more crucial edge over test tubes and unprotected culture medium in open dishes. It dramatically increased the time he could keep the embryo outside its incubator safely—long enough for him to perform experimental microsurgery. Research laboratories commonly used the mineral oil. Most clinical units did not. They said it was too messy. "People were afraid to use it," said Mina Alikani. "I was afraid." Anything that complicated the lab routine increased the chance that the technicians would make a mistake.

The difference in technique was typical of the inconsistencies in procedure from lab to lab. After questioning 160 U.S. embryo laboratories in 1990, the General Accounting Office, the investigative arm of Congress, found dramatic disagreements in the lab techniques used to help childless couples conceive—and an even wider variation in how often the labs were able to get their patients pregnant. Part of the reason was the age and health of the men and women themselves. But the variations also were due to the different lab methods. With no accepted clinical "cookbook" to guide them, IVF practitioners improvised freely.

There were so many cooks, so many broths. Some labs kept

their bottles of culture medium for as long as a month before refreshing the stock; others mixed a fresh stock every week. Some laboratories incubated the eggs barely an hour before inseminating them; others waited up to eight hours. One-third of the laboratories inseminated the eggs only once. Some labs kept the resulting embryos in lab dishes for less than a day; one in five laboratories cultured the embryos for as long as 60 hours. Some transferred no more than three embryos at a time to a woman's womb; others five. One even transferred 12 at a time. The humidity levels in the embryo incubators ranged from high desert to tropical rainforest.

In the United States, the American Fertility Society—the one major professional society in a position to insist that infertility specialists adopt uniform quality controls—had been reluctant to do so. The only national register of laboratory success rates was kept by a drug company. States exempted the labs from standard medical regulations. Even federal standards would be useless without the will to enforce them.

The problem transcended national borders. In England, medical societies ruthlessly censured any infertility specialist who violated the British voluntary code of practice. By 1991, Parliament made violation of its licensing code regulating laboratory conception a crime punishable by up to 10 years in prison. The Australian Fertility Society also adopted rigid laboratory guidelines, but had no way to enforce them. The first time it tried to impose sanctions against one of its members for failing to adhere to the new standards, the clinic director sued. The doctor who filed suit had been the head of the committee that had formulated the rules.

"The guidelines were just old-boy stuff," said Dr. Douglas M. Saunders, a former president of the Australian society. "There were no teeth."

Dr. Bryan Hudson, chairman of the regulatory committee, said he learned the hard way how reluctant his colleagues were to enforce standards. "They are a bunch of bloody wimps," he said.

Even as a temporary womb, the plastic lab dish wasn't worth much. Despite 20 years of research with human embryos, scientists still had only a glimmer of what it took to nurture an embryo properly. In Cohen's laboratory at RBA, only about one in 10 laboratory embryos developed all the way to birth. Nationally, the figure was about three in 100. "That's a terrible waste of embryos," Cohen said.

The embryologists tinkered incessantly with the lab conditions. They were working blind, trying to duplicate an environment they had never really seen and could never directly explore. When they tried something new, they had only the most indirect evidence of its success. To boost their pregnancy rates, clinics routinely transferred several embryos into a woman's womb. If the woman became pregnant, the embryologist had no way to determine which embryo had survived.

They had remarkably little to guide them in diagnosing the health and vigor of the sperm, eggs, and embryos they manipulated. Basic research with laboratory animals could only explain so much about human reproduction. The human egg, for instance, can be fertilized for up to 32 hours. The egg of the mouse, most commonly used in laboratory research, cannot be fertilized after about two hours. Nothing could compare to the promiscuity of the zona-free hamster egg, which allowed itself to be penetrated by the sperm of just about any mammalian species. "No animal is a good model for another species," said research embryologist Carol Keefer. "The mouse is not a model for the human. If you want to learn about a species, you have to work with that species."

In Cohen's laboratory, the human eggs and embryos received unusual scrutiny. Cohen and his assistants photographed and videotaped them. They freeze-framed, magnified, and enhanced the pictures in the hopes that some standard characteristics of health and quality would emerge.

To improve survival rates, researchers in Australia experimented with growth fluids. At Royal North Shore Hospital in Sydney, embryologist Chris O'Neill doubled the clinic's pregnancy rate by seasoning the medium with a body chemical called platelet-activating factor. At the University of Melbourne, embryologist Alexander Lopata mixed in vitamins and amino acids. The embryos became more robust. At the Jones Institute in Norfolk, researchers collected immature eggs from patients, fertilized them, then monitored them for clues to development. Still, too many embryos died, and no one knew why.

Cohen took a different approach. If no one could explain the chemistry of the human womb well enough to duplicate it, he would construct an artificial womb in the laboratory. He let natural fetal "helper" cells do the manual labor. He farmed many of his embryos on a bed of fetal cow cells salvaged from the slaughterhouse.

It seemed to work. The embryos grew faster, seemed more robust, displayed fewer signs of fragmentation. Even a day on the fetal cells improved the health of embryos. The pregnancy rate per patient increased by 10 percent. The miscarriage rate was lower. By May 1990, 35 women had delivered healthy babies from the treated embryos. Cohen had lifted the idea from cattle breeders who had been doing it for years.

"We don't really hardly culture cow embryos anymore in a medium alone because it just doesn't work nearly as well," said Klaus Wiemer, a cattle embryologist at Alta-Genetics in Calgary, Canada, who developed the experiment with Cohen. "It's almost become obsolete. These fetal cells have recently been shown to provide the best support for early-stage cattle embryos, sheep embryos, and goat embryos. If it works better in these domesticated species, why wouldn't it work better in a human?"

It was not a new question, but Cohen and Wiemer were the first to use human embryos to answer it. In France, researchers had been equally anxious to perform the same experiments, but a national ethics commission held up their work for three years. In Australia, researchers at the Monash University Centre for Early Human Development experimented with human fetal tissue as a growth bed for mouse embryos. But they had never been given permission to try it with human embryos.

"They can do it now because we broke the ice," Wiemer said. "When our paper came out showing that it works, that broke the ice for a lot of other people."

Their success was suggestive. Scientists considered parking human embryos in the wombs of rabbits or sheep temporarily.

The developing embryos could be safely stored in the mammal's womb and then flushed from the animal several days later. The idea was not farfetched. Cattle breeders had been known to ship an entire herd of prize purebred cows to Europe inside the womb of a rabbit. Although no one had ever proposed trying it with human embryos, several countries had already passed laws to forbid placing a human embryo in an animal.

Researchers in Louisiana, however, toyed with an alternative. They tried growing sheep and goat embryos in hen's eggs. When they tucked the embryonic livestock into the egg's amniotic sac, it consistently promoted embryonic growth. There was no apparent reason why it would not work equally well with human embryos.

Before entering Cohen's Atlanta laboratory, Wiemer slipped blue-paper covers over his brown cowboy boots and ambled into the laboratory. His walk had been shaped by his high-school hobby—rodeo bull-riding. He checked the embryos in their beds of fetal cells, then punched the image of one embryo up on the video screen. Its four cells looked like helium balloons ready to burst.

"It is the champagne of culture medium. Look at them. They are intoxicated," he said. "They are drinking Cohen champagne."

Mina Alikani, visiting from Cornell to study Cohen's laboratory techniques, also examined the screen. "It's a nice, clean-looking embryo. Beautiful. It has the potential to be the next Miss Georgia," she said.

Wiemer shook his head emphatically. "He is going to be another Robert Redford."

She looked at him coolly. "Why do you assume she is male? We'll see in nine months," she said.

The early embryo on the screen literally took after its mother. As it fertilized, reorganized, and split into new cells, it followed a pattern set in motion before the egg from which it developed ever left its mother's ovary. Not until it reached the four-cell stage would the growing embryo actually incorporate its father's genes to produce its own unique genetic structure. The new genes only switched on once the embryo had grown into eight cells. The quality of the human egg was, therefore, paramount because it controlled the embryo's early development.

Often by the time a surgeon siphoned the egg from the ovary, the damage had already been done. To avoid such complications, Cohen insisted on supervising the hormone injections used to stimulate the production of eggs. The doctors considered it their own medical preserve. They often clashed with Cohen.

"Who is the reproductive endocrinologist here?" the doctors would say. "You or me?"

"How can you deal with eggs and embryos if you don't know how they were made? How can you make eggs if you don't know how they are going to be used?" Cohen would protest. "If you don't do the follicular stimulation right, you won't get pregnancies. If you don't do the embryo transfer gently, you won't get pregnancies, either," he said. "That subject is really difficult to bring up with doctors because it is so personal."

He insisted on bringing it up, anyway. The doctors were proud of their touch, and they generally considered Cohen a pain. He was like the neighbor who keeps nagging the cook not to slam the kitchen door while the cake is rising.

In the name of quality control, many labs strove for a single, regimented routine. Cohen, however, tailored his treatments as closely as possible to the patient under his microscope. The lab conditions and hormone treatments often differed from month to month. The embryos' survival rates were unpredictable. The embryologists rarely consulted patients about changes in culture medium or other matters of laboratory technique, even though each adjustment could significantly alter their chances of becoming pregnant. And, if patients chose to join in Cohen's controlled clinical experiments, they had no way to ensure their embryos would receive the most advanced treatment.

"If you tell patients about all the variations, you will be talking to them all day long," Cohen said, irritated. "My feeling is they can agree not to do this at all or they can leave it up to the specialist." He checked his anger and shook his head. "In a way we are bullshitting them. We tell them the truth about everything except the embryos. We always tell them the embryos are wonderful. We bullshit them."

Cohen ran down the list of experiments and double-checked the consent forms. On the couple's master medical sheet, the boxes had been plainly marked. Partial zona dissection, yes. Embryo hatching, yes. Co-culture on fetal cow cells, no. Enucleation to remove any extra pronucleus, yes.

Embryo freezing.

Of all the consent forms Lisa and Bill Fagg signed for Jacques Cohen, they had lingered longest over the permission to freeze their extra embryos. The few mimeographed pages struck directly at the heart of their faith in the future, at the strength of their marriage and the value they placed on the human embryos they would create. This was different from the other experiments for which they had volunteered. Embryo freezing was not designed to enhance the survival of an individual embryo. It was designed to sidestep the ethical problems posed by too many embryos. "There is a kind of moral obligation to freeze," said Graham Wright. "You have to do something with the extra embryos."

The embryo cell freezer—a squat, gray, wheezing mechanical contrivance—was a time machine. It arrested an embryo's development in a bubbling bath of liquid nitrogen and effectively hurled it into the future. Couples conceived a litter of embryos, froze them, then doled them into the womb a few at a time, often resulting in fraternal twins born years apart. One Australian woman gave birth to two babies two years apart who had been conceived at the same time and then frozen. In 1989—five years after the birth of the first—she was pregnant with a third thawed from the same set. All three embryos were created in the same moment, but the first would start school before the third was actually born. Nobody really knew how long an embryo could stay safely in cold storage, but it was long enough at least to outlive the marriages that produced them or the men and women themselves. There seemed no theoretical limit.

Frozen embryos forced couples and courts to reconsider the

nature of pregnancy and parenthood. For potential parents, it was uncharted psychological territory only superficially covered by consent forms. Clauses covered death, menopause, adoption, and, belatedly, divorce. They made no provision for emotional exhaustion or personal bankruptcy. Nor did they consider the possibility that the clinic itself might go out of business or its skilled embryologists quit. The embryos could outlast the memory of the techniques by which they were frozen. Thus, the new technology created new heartaches.

Courtroom battles raged over custody of frozen embryos. The courtroom struggle of one refrigerator technician and his infertile wife became a tabloid fable of the new technology. When Junior Davis, thirty-one, and Mary Sue Davis, twenty-nine, fell in love in West Germany, their only intention was to marry in their Ohio hometown, settle down, and raise a family. Instead, their marriage ended in divorce. Their last days together were spent in a Tennessee courtroom fighting for possession of the only family they were ever able to conceive: seven human embryos frozen in liquid nitrogen at a Knoxville infertility clinic during 1988. They had never signed a legally binding consent form in which husband and wife agreed in advance on the disposition of their frozen progeny. "I am the mother of these embryos," Mary Sue Davis told a rapt courtroom audience. "They are the beginning of life. I consider them my children. The only person who has a right to bear them is me. They are a part of me and they belong in my body." When she won the right to bear them, her husband protested that his reproductive rights had been "raped." Yet she had lost something, too. A few months later, she announced that she would put the embryos up for anonymous adoption.

Both remarried, but neither could escape the emotional power the clusters of frozen cells exercised over their lives. Junior Davis vowed to seek custody if the embryos were ever allowed to grow into children, no matter whose womb served to quicken them. As the litigation and appeals dragged on, an attorney volunteered to serve as legal guardian to oversee the seven frozen embryos. In 1990, a three-member appeals panel overturned the custody order because it violated the father's constitutional right not to procreate, and granted the estranged couple joint control of the seven embryos. Judge Herschel P. Franks said that "it would be repugnant and offensive to constitutional principals to order Mary Sue to implant these fertilized ova against her will. . . . It would be equally repugnant to order Junior to bear the psychological, if not the legal, consequences of paternity against his will." The ruling left the ex-husband and the ex-wife where they began, with seven frozen embryos and no idea what to do with them.

The longer embryos lingered in frozen storage, the more likely it was that they would become subject to divorce actions. Kort, Massey, and Elsner at Reproductive Biology Associates knew it was only a matter of time before some of the embryos in their care became the innocent bystanders in divorce court. The letter, when it came, carried the return address of a small Alabama law firm. Writing on behalf of an irate husband, the lawyer advised the clinic that two fertilized human eggs at RBA had become part of a divorce proceeding. The client "demands that neither of these eggs be released to anyone, especially his wife." The lawyer tried to be polite. "We are not threatening you in this letter, but merely letting you know the situation as it now stands between the parties." For infertility specialists, divorce had become another occupational hazard.

Bill and Lisa Fagg had spread the consent forms out on the dining room table and read them again and again. She was grateful that she had to make her mind up now. "I still am very confused about the whole issue, but I wouldn't want the dilemma next year or ten years from now of having to decide what to do with them," she said.

"We read every page twenty times. We talked about it for hours. If Bill died tomorrow, he would want me to have those children. We would make an effort to have the frozen embryos as children. If we didn't use them, I wouldn't want them destroyed. I don't think I would want them used for scientific research. There's a possibility that they might be allowed to be born and I don't like the doctors experimenting on that. I'd want to donate them to a couple."

Susan and David Parr were uncomfortable with the idea of another couple raising their offspring. They gave Jacques

Cohen permission to experiment with any embryos they did not use themselves. "We could donate them, but I don't necessarily trust other people to be good parents to my embryos," she said. "Let's face it, that's as close as I've gotten to children. To me these embryos are life, emotionally. They are not my babies yet, but they are my embryos. Maybe by experimenting on them, they can come up with something. That would be worth it to me to save some people from having to go through this."

Divorce. Death. Custody. Adoption. The couples were making a will for children they would never have.

"As far as the embryos were concerned," David Boone recalled, "our attitude was that if we are alive and together, we can have them as babies. But if we aren't, they can do whatever they want with them for medical science purposes or for education. We didn't go through any great agony. I don't have a problem with the fact that someone may look at them under a microscope and pull them apart with needles and pins for scientific purposes."

Bill and Lisa Fagg signed up. And in August, Cohen froze five embryos for them. Most laboratories froze embryos in plastic straws. Cohen enclosed each embryo inside its own handmade glass ampule. He sealed it in the flame of a propane blowtorch. If he held it too long in the flame, the embryo could boil. If the ampule was improperly sealed, it would, when thawed, explode like a firecracker.

Mina Alikani watched the blue flame turn yellow and the tip of the glass ampule turn cherry red. "This scares me more than anything else," she said, "this flame and the embryo so near it."

Physically, the five embryos could survive as long as the flask that held them. Atlanta would agree to store a frozen embryo for no more than a decade. Norfolk would keep them for no more than six years. In England, by law, a clinic could keep frozen embryos for no more than five years. "Whether we like it or not, some of these embryos will be stored indefinitely," Cohen said. When the time limit expired, few clinics would have the nerve to destroy the embryos in their custody without permission. And no matter how many consent forms a couple may have signed, some couples would change their minds.

The social dilemmas stemmed from a scientific solution to the most troubling technical and moral failure of laboratory conception—excess embryos. Couples who had worked so hard to conceive suddenly found themselves with too much of a good thing. Women undergoing laboratory conception ended up bearing unusually large numbers of twins, triplets, and quadruplets that threatened the health of the women who carried them. Often, they were forced to deliver by caesarean section. The children themselves suffered hardships in the crowded womb; they were more likely to be born premature or underweight. At the University of Sydney, in Australia, Dr. Paul Lancaster determined that the perinatal death rate of IVF babies was almost five times that of the national average.

Some clinics offered selective abortion, called fetal reduction, so that women could reduce the fetuses they were carrying to a more manageable number. Quadruplets became twins. Triplets became a single child.

Between 1985 and 1988, a medical team at the Thomas Jefferson University Hospital in Philadelphia, which pioneered the technique, successfully performed selective abortions on 46 women carrying three or more fetuses, in the hopes that they could increase the chance that one healthy child would be born. Writing in the medical journal *Lancet*, the doctors said, "For people who accord little or no moral status to the fetus, our indications for a reduction of multifetal pregnancies are ethically justified as a function of the woman's right to control the disposition of her pregnancy. This approach will be troublesome, however, for people who accord substantial moral status to the fetus as a living, developing human being."

Even when such infants were carried safely to term, their sheer numbers could create a financial burden for the parents who raised them. One Michigan mother conceived quintuplets through in vitro fertilization. She brought them home one and two at a time so her family could get over the shock. An Australian woman, known publicly only as Marie, had been implanted with four embryos at the Concept clinic in Perth. To her dismay, she found herself bearing quadruplets. She demanded that three of the embryos be aborted. Her surgeons refused. When she delivered, Marie and her husband put three of the four babies up for adoption. They said they could not face the financial and emotional burden of quadruplets. When their decision became public, they found they couldn't face the outraged public opinion, either. To keep the family intact, the local government volunteered money and counseling.

When human embryo freezing was achieved in 1984, clinics seized gratefully on the procedure. It allowed them to reduce the odds of a multiple pregnancy by transferring fewer embryos. It made the IVF procedure easier on the woman by eliminating the need for repeated rounds of hormone injections and egg-retrieval surgery. They argued, too, that the womb was more receptive when it was not irritated by the fertility drugs. Doctors said that cold storage also would spare embryos the rigors of extended development outside the body. So, to the risks of growth in an artificial womb, they added the risks of freezing and thawing. Barely 60 percent of the embryos would survive. Those that did were said to be hardier and more likely to survive a pregnancy. With little fanfare, researchers had added the ability to withstand a cell freezer to the list of human survival characteristics. They made an evolutionary virtue of laboratory necessity.

Within five years, clinics had filled thousands of containers with frozen embryos racked in metal tubes out of sight and largely out of mind. For both parents and practitioners, the frozen embryos were a lien on the future.

"We are one generation of people that has decided, for better or for worse, to create banks of frozen embryos," said Anibal Acosta at Norfolk, where hundreds were in suspended animation. "We have said that these embryos are going to be kept in there for the reproductive life of the mother. Some of those mothers are twenty-five years of age. Then you are committing yourself to keeping those embryos for twenty years. And in twenty years' time, we will have retired. A new generation is going to come here to take over. They will find a bank with maybe thousands of embryos. Are they responsible for that? Who is going to be responsible for those embryos in the next generation?"

Before coming to Atlanta, Graham Wright and Jacques Cohen had collaborated briefly at a clinic in Barcelona, Spain, where they froze embryos for 50 couples. The clinic later suspended operations. "There are frozen embryos stuck there," Wright said. "They are the property of the clinic—at least they are their responsibility. Is anybody topping them up with liquid nitrogen every week? I don't know. Do they remember to do it? I don't even want to call to find out."

Lisa Fagg addressed Christmas cards. She hoped it might take her mind off waiting. There were still days yet before a blood test could determine whether she was pregnant. She paged through her address book. "There are people you talk to once a year in Christmas cards. I thought: 'Well, what have we done this year?' We've gone through infertility treatments. When you think about it, that's all we've done all year," she said.

She ticked off the calendar on her fingers.

"We went through a cycle last October. We were going to go through it again in January, but Bill got sick. We went through one in April, went through one in October. Really, we've gone from one cycle almost right into another continuously." She shook her head ruefully. "There are only so many times you can get your arm drawn for blood and have your rear end stuck with a needle and have your legs and everything else stuck before you have to walk away from it for a little while. If this works, I'll be ecstatic. If it doesn't, it will be a long time before I go through another full cycle. I'm not even real concerned about the embryos we still have frozen. I want a rest. I need a break from it," she said.

If she was pregnant, she would never have to go back. She could put the five frozen embryos up for adoption. If she had to return, she could wait until she could rebuild her courage. She had time. The frozen embryos had been in storage four months. They could wait another year or two. She rocked in the sun-room and tried to picture the embryos inside her.

When it finally came, the telephone call telling her she had again failed to become pregnant would be devastating. "Now I have thirteen babies in heaven," she would say. And five on ice.

4

Swimming Against the Current

Only a few sperm were moving, twitching fitfully like tadpoles in the mud of an evaporating rain puddle. Some were stuck together in clumps. Some had two heads. Others shivered with palsy. Between them were whitish flecks of debris and dead cells. Bathed in the green glow on the microscope stage, the abnormal sperm cells looked like the casualties of biochemical warfare.

The cells were so damaged that the computer could not recognize them or count them electronically. Cohen turned away from the microscope and quickly punched a number on the telephone. The husband and wife were waiting together down the hall. They had already spent thousands of dollars preparing for this day. She had taken hormone injections for weeks to force her ovaries to produce extra eggs. She was scheduled for surgery in an hour. Cohen canceled it.

"There are no motile sperm," he said into the receiver. "This sample cannot fertilize. That's the story." He hung up. "We should have canceled this a long time ago. But the patient wanted to go through with it," he said. It was a doctor's job to break the news to them face to face.

In Shakespeare's day, most people believed that, curled inside each sperm, there was a preformed person, a homunculus, who took root and grew inside a woman's womb. Beliefs had changed only slightly in the centuries since. Until recently, almost nothing was known about the causes of male infertility, and remarkably little systematic research had been conducted on its treatment. Fetal defects caused by abnormal sperm were often blamed on maternal age instead.

Compared to the techniques developed to manipulate the female reproductive system, treatments for male infertility were primitive at best. "Efforts on prevention and treatment are largely guesswork," congressional investigators noted. In the United States, the quality of the average sperm sample had been steadily dropping for decades, but nobody knew why, or seemed to care.

While researchers were consumed by the problems of the female reproductive system, most were baffled by men. Among almost half of the married couples who had trouble conceiving, the man was the infertile partner. But almost always, the woman ended up as the patient. To diagnose and treat male infertility effectively, doctors had to overcome their own social prejudices as well as the scientific obstacles. Finally, they were forced to confront the other half of the human equation.

Given the importance society placed on paternity and on sperm, the reluctance to treat male infertility is puzzling. Modern commentators have looked no further than the sex of the researchers themselves, who are overwhelmingly male, for an explanation. Masculine pride was too vulnerable to admit any procreative failure; any failure to conceive must always be the woman's fault, they suggested. Men were traditionally reluctant even to consider the possibility they were at fault or to seek a doctor's help for anything involving their ability to procreate. Women, on the other hand, long ago got used to the idea that their reproductive organs were the object of constant medical analysis. Doctors, for example, have long been alert to the fact that certain chemicals can damage fetuses developing in a woman's womb, but they only recently have considered the possibility that dangerous chemicals in a man's body may cause subtle defects in sperm that could, in turn, lead to birth defects. Feminist analysts soundly argue that the lack of research and treatment into male infertility is one more example of the preferential workings of a male-dominated medical establishment intent on preserving reproductive control.

A close examination of the technology suggests that infertile men have been equally victimized. In the earliest and most successful forms of assisted reproduction, doctors cured male infertility with an act of male medical aggression—by simply eliminating the husband as a physical reproductive partner.

Artificial insemination was so easy that about 172,000 women in the United States tried it at least once every year. It was so profitable that 11,000 doctors offered the procedure, charging in total about $163 million annually. In all, women who conceived through artificial insemination with their husband's sperm gave birth to about 35,000 children every year. Women who were inseminated with a donor's sperm gave birth to another 30,000 children annually.

Long before anyone dared to freeze an embryo, frozen semen was cheap and readily available. It could be frozen in five minutes and stored safely for at least five years. The practice became so common that, in 1991, U.S. troops leaving for frontline duty in the Persian Gulf placed frozen sperm in storage so that, if they were killed in action, their wives could still conceive and bear their children. The freezing process sharply curtailed its ability to fertilize, but donor sperm was so plentiful that nobody cared. Sperm banks published donor catalogs and offered premium "lines" that promised to make a woman pregnant two months sooner than less-expensive semen. When the first commercial sperm bank in the U.S. opened in 1970, it hoped to profit from the second thoughts of the 600,000 men who had vasectomies every year. Increasing male infertility and the advent of AIDS increased a booming business because only a large-scale commercial enterprise seemed willing to invest the time and testing equipment needed to ensure that donor semen was free of the lethal virus. One clinic's sales climbed from $500 a month in 1976 to $30,000 a decade later. Couples could reserve a donor in advance to ensure that all their children would be genetically related "full" siblings. At medical conventions, the sperm banks drummed up business by handing out T-shirts that advertised "future people."

The first woman to conceive through donor insemination never knew that she bore a stranger's son. Neither did her husband. The woman sought help at a Philadelphia hospital in 1884 to learn why she was childless. The examining doctor determined that she was fertile but her husband was not. Then, in front of six medical students, he anesthetized her and injected her with a rubber syringe full of sperm contributed by a medical student. The medical team found it such an interesting experiment that they reported it in a medical journal. It apparently never occurred to any of them to seek the couple's consent or even explain what they were doing.

In the decades following the experiment, the use of donor sperm raised such hackles that states like Ohio considered making everyone involved—doctor, donor, husband, and wife—subject to criminal fines and imprisonment. Married women who used donor sperm to conceive were, in many countries, guilty of adultery, even if the husbands had consented to the procedure. Any child so conceived was a bastard whose legal status concerning inheritance and support was uncertain at best. Well into the 1960s, there were U.S. judges willing to rule that, regardless of the husband's consent, the wife who used donor sperm to conceive had committed an act of infidelity. Instead of effective medical treatment, infertile men eventually got legal reform. By 1986, U.S. lawmakers in 31 states had revised the biological definition of fatherhood. The laws abstracted paternity. Fatherhood became a social, not a sexual, act. The legal husband who consented to the use of donor sperm became the father of the child. Seventeen states specifically stated that sperm donors have no parental rights. At least one Oregon state-appeals court, however, ruled such blanket prohibitions unconstitutional.

Only belatedly did the medical profession acknowledge the emotional risks of the procedure. Decades after it became routine, the American Fertility Society warned its members to give "careful consideration" to alerting any woman and her partner about the psychological risks of donor insemination. The doctors were urged to offer counseling and, if possible, treat any male infertility problem before resorting to artificial insemination.

However damaging psychologically, artificial insemination and the use of donor sperm were so simple technically, and sperm so plentiful, that there seemed little scientific incentive to pursue alternatives.

Nature is profligate with human sperm. Sperm cells, produced by the millions, are earnest commuters in a rush-hour traffic jam, their heads packed to bursting with tightly coiled genetic messages. Sperm cells are so hardy they can withstand 1,100 times the force of gravity—70 times more than the human body itself can survive. They live on sugar like voracious adolescents consuming candy bars. They are so energetic that in six hours the microscopic wrigglers can swim a meter. And they are as dumb as a post. "Sperm will try to inseminate air bubbles," one clinician explained. By contrast, the human egg is so prized by nature that only one is produced at a time. The egg is larger than any other cell and is physically arresting to view; it is fragile, inaccessible, discriminating, mysterious in its workings. Intricate and subtle, it enfolds and nurtures. It would be hard to imagine two more stereotypical sexual tissues.

More important for the prestige of medical practitioners, the act of egg retrieval is a matter of surgically elegant manipulation. To stimulate and obtain human eggs is to control the seat of conception and fetal development. To manipulate embryos is to cultivate the bud of human life. It requires advanced training, dexterity, and scientific skill.

By contrast, sperm is obtained by masturbation. Many clinics put the husbands in a bathroom or a "masturbatorium" with a tattered copy of *Playboy* or *Penthouse*. Even among those most dedicated to the diagnosis and correction of infertility problems, for whom human sexuality should most clearly be a matter of organic chemistry and cell biology, there was often the unconscious attitude that the male patients were not quite "real men." In the laboratory, potency became a matter of measurable sperm counts, motility, and the ability of sperm to penetrate a hamster egg. At the same time, male sexual sensitivities were rarely spared.

"Oh, well, men can just do it anywhere," said one woman responsible for analyzing the sperm samples at one of the country's largest IVF clinics. "They tell you they can't, but they can."

Thus, many of the men forced to seek a stranger's help in conception were equally the victims of medical technology and sexual stereotyping. For infertile women, the marriage bed became an operating table. For men, it became a toilet seat or an armchair in the "jack room." Like the women, they juggled rage and shame with a helpless faith in technology. Many of them realized that, as men, they were not even considered an interesting research project. Milked of their gametes, they felt dehumanized.

"I have an emotional reaction when a young nurse hands me a cup for a sperm sample. You bring back your pitiful sperm and then it gets injected as if you aren't strong enough to do it yourself. One nurse put it under a microscope and started telling me how lousy it was," said one medical professional in Virginia who underwent six years of unsuccessful treatments for his infertility. "It was," he said slowly, "an awkward social situation." He and his wife finally adopted.

Other men felt equally abashed when producing sperm samples for lab tests or fertilization. "I always felt like the man in the trench coat who is about to expose himself," one man said.

Another man added, "There were times I just couldn't do it. I'd kill a two-thousand-dollar procedure because I couldn't do it."

A third infertile man said flatly of himself, "This thing you have to pump up to give a sperm sample is a piece of junk."

In the clinics, the staff could feel the tension. "The dynamic on Saturdays when the husbands are there is terrible. When the problem is one hundred percent male factor, there can be a very intense, terrifying husband," said Catharine Kruithoff at Norfolk.

At Reproductive Biology Associates in Atlanta, almost one in every four couples involved an infertile man. Carlene Elsner saw them in her office every day. "Her husband has no sperm. He feels castrated because he's been told he can't have a child. She is angry because she has to use donor sperm. There is a lot of free-floating hostility," she said.

For most men, even a limited foray into reproductive medicine left them on completely alien ground. "Men don't easily accept people messing around with their private parts. Women go through it more. Men are not socialized into this. There are many fears and issues that men have about another man evaluating their private parts," said one Washington, D.C., psychologist who had been treated unsuccessfully for infertility. "There is a certain amount of sexual performance demanded of a man just to be tested. You don't lie on a table and get looked at. Masturbation is an emotionally significant thing. The hundredth time you give a sample, it becomes a very dehumanizing thing, very mechanical. It's hard to confront the feeling of helplessness and the feeling you are out of control."

He recalled a married couple who sought his professional counsel because the husband had been repeatedly unfaithful. The husband was infertile. He told the psychologist his sexual infidelity was meaningless because "nothing could come of it." Biologically barren, the husband was convinced that even betrayal had been robbed of its meaning, that he was a sexual cipher.

In Boston, one man discussed the failure of his marriage to produce children for two hours without mentioning that, like his wife, he had a physical disability that affected his fertility. When he finally volunteered the information, his voice trembled with anger. "They take your stuff and her stuff and they do whatever they want with it. They tell you your stuff is dead. You realize that what matters is this technique they've been practicing for twenty years under a microscope. That's what matters—their technique. And you are strictly the meat." He had been trying to conceive with his wife for eight years. "I can fertilize an egg but I can't make a baby." By the time he reached the end of his last sentence, he was almost shouting. His fist hit the table. He looked surprised. "I'm starting to get wild," he said.

To fertilize a human egg, a man normally releases between 40 million and 200 million sperm cells. His sperm count changes with the seasons; higher in the winter, lower in the summer. Only one sperm cell, however, is actually needed to penetrate the egg and trigger fertilization. A horse produces from four billion to nine billion sperm. The pig releases as many as 20 billion sperm. Other species are more sparing. The honeybee releases an average of 20 to 30 sperm per egg. The queen fire ant, which mates only once in its life, husbands three sperm to fertilize each of its thousands of eggs.

Each human sperm cell takes about two months to mature. Scientists do not know precisely how to detect a healthy one. They still aren't sure why, when nature is so miserly in releasing one mature human egg each month, it requires the production of so many millions of sperm cells. Perhaps human reproduction is built around the idea that human sperm are inherently defective. Most infertile men do not have enough sperm, or have sperm that are misshapen or that do not move properly. They may not be able to fertilize an egg because they cannot penetrate the egg's cover.

"Human reproduction is terribly inefficient. If we were bulls, we'd have all been shot long ago," said Dr. Peter Braude, a leading infertility specialist at Cambridge University.

The sperm cell is not capable of fertilizing an egg until it swims free of the semen that transports it and is chemically conditioned by the fluids in the female tract. Some men and women are allergic to sperm; the interaction of cells and body fluids designed to activate the sperm instead kills it. Their immune systems produce antibodies that cling to the head, neck, or tail of the sperm and hinder its ability to penetrate the egg. Their bodies react as if the swimming cells are invading disease bacteria. Indeed, semen is so often a source of infection that lab technicians routinely inoculate the culture dishes with antibiotics.

Once researchers started investigating human sperm cells, they found no shortage of problems. Every man carries some sperm with flawed chromosomes—even those who have no history of inherited disease. Common medications like sulfa drugs are toxic to sperm. Nicotine, caffeine, and cigarette-smoking affect its quality. Electromagnetic fields and ultrasound waves also impair male reproductive cells. The testicles, hanging free of the body to maintain the sperm at 94 or 95 degrees Fahrenheit, readily absorb pesticides and other hazardous chemicals. Even relatively minor increases in heat—as little as a degree for a prolonged period—can impair sperm quality. Most of the time, however, the doctors never figured out the problem. To assess the sperm's fertility, they did little more than count the number of cells and determine their ability to swim. Clinical diagnostic techniques are incapable of detecting numerous molecular abnormalities or functional defects.

"A man's ability to produce healthy sperm is basically trashed by the facts of modern living," said Henry Malter.

Lab technicians routinely concentrated the sperm. One sperm bank's premium service offered twice as many sperm cells per sample—a kind of higher human octane.

The image of Lisa Fagg's egg rolled across the monitor screen—a translucent, elongated oval. The egg was one of 11 she had produced during her third attempt at pregnancy in August 1989. Dozens of sperm clung to the enormous cell. Although everything about her husband's sperm tested normally, the barrier around her egg proved impenetrable. Compared to other species, the zona membrane around the human egg is particularly thick, rigid, and difficult to penetrate. Perhaps the artificial hormones had made this one even more brittle.

The embryologists could make her ovaries produce multiple eggs on demand and ripen them like fruit. They could give her eggs donated by other women, in a female version of artificial insemination. They could enhance and concentrate the healthiest sperm her husband's body could produce. They were still learning, however, how to force a union between the two.

To help an infertile couple like Bill and Lisa, Cohen didn't have to understand why the egg and sperm had failed to meld. He could give the sperm a physical boost—a leg up over the wall of the zona membrane. With a glass needle, he made a passage for the sperm to enter. He inserted the needle into the egg and then massaged it until the egg dropped off.

"The sperm still have to find the hole. It is microscopic billiards," Cohen said.

In his hands, the operation appeared deceptively easy. Whatever objections nature had to the union, Cohen had overcome them; the eggs fertilized. A day later, Lisa Fagg came to the clinic. He placed the embryos in her uterus. They did not survive. When she returned in November for her fourth round of experimental procedures, only two eggs out of 13 fertilized. They did not survive, either. He could make the eggs fertilize, but he could not make them implant in her womb.

There were risks with the zona-drilling procedure. The acid used by one lab to drill holes in the egg inhibited embryo development. The eggs themselves could be damaged by rough handling. Once the barrier was breached, many sperm could enter—not just the one that nature intended. The result was an abnormal embryo that, in a sense, contained the genetic inheritance from three sources—the egg and two or more sperm. And the healthier the sperm, the more severe the problem.

Up to half the embryos resulting from egg surgery were genetically abnormal. The labs discarded them or froze them to save for other experiments. The microsurgery caused as many problems as it solved. It was, like so many things in laboratory conception, only better than nothing. While Cohen cleared a passage for the sperm to enter, other doctors tried to inject mechanically a single sperm cell directly into the center of the egg. At the Jones Institute in Norfolk, doctors performed the experiment with several dozen couples.

"These were people who had maybe five sluggishly motile sperm on a slide, instead of five million," said Lucinda Veeck, the institute's senior embryologist. They transferred embryos into 14 volunteers; none became pregnant. "Our concern is that we could be overriding the natural selection process by injecting an abnormal sperm," Veeck said. "On our consent form, there is a paragraph that notes that, as far as risks, there is so little information that the risks are unknown."

When they injected the sperm directly into the tissue of the egg itself, researchers tried to immobilize it without actually killing it. Some researchers injected freeze-dried sperm. Others shaved off the sperm membrane, cut off its tail, and injected

the tightly coiled bundle of male genetic material that remained. Researchers working with laboratory animals quickly
discovered that both techniques caused genetic abnormalities.

"You really have to come up with another trick," Jacques
Cohen said.

What he really wanted was something more precise and less
destructive—to insert a single sperm into the empty space
between the egg and its outer membrane. Throughout the
winter of 1989–90, his team at Cornell experimented with
mouse eggs to craft the proper tools and techniques needed
to inject a single cell without killing the egg or the sperm.
They brooded over the risk of undetectable genetic damage.
The proper name for the procedure was "subzonal insertion."
Cohen, Malter, and Talansky dubbed their experimental technique "schlepping." It was driving them crazy.

"Even if you do the sperm injection perfectly, you could still
not get fertilization," said Malter. "I have very little faith in
it. There can be so many things wrong with sperm that you
can't see. There are cases where we don't know what else to
do. These people may have only four sperm. Maybe we should
tell them to go to an adoption agency."

Halfway around the world, at the Centre for Early Human
Development in Melbourne, Australia, Alan Trounson's embryo research group already had perfected the sperm injection
technique. It had been part of their laboratory routine for almost five years, but local laws regulating embryo research
blocked them from trying it in human beings.

So frustrated had they become at local regulatory delays that
in 1988 they finally crossed the state border to Sydney, in New
South Wales, to conduct their key human embryo experiments
in another jurisdiction. They exported their research, putting
themselves beyond the law.

At his lab bench in Melbourne, Danny Sakkis trapped a
single wriggling sperm in the hollow of a beveled-glass needle
and lifted it into the air. The sperm batted against the walls
of the hair-thin tube like a fly in a jar.

With a second needle, placed in a small black-plastic canister
the size of a spool of thread, Sakkis took hold of an egg. He

lined up the two under the microscope and then injected the sperm in the cavity under the egg's outer membrane. In the narrow space, the sperm swam restlessly, its tail lashing against the outer sheath.

To make the sperm and eggs more easily visible under the microscope, Sakkis heightened the colors electronically. The sperm droplet turned sky blue. The egg drop was peach. The egg itself was crazed at its edges with rainbow hues like an oil slick. His tools were glowing slivers of glass. To the naked eye, it was a watery smear on a slide. Through the eyepiece, it looked as if Sakkis were dissecting the sunset.

Sakkis rotated the egg to show off the sperm swimming inside. "The sperm swim around quite happily once they are in there," he said. He leaned back from the gray Olympus microscope and the two Leitz micromanipulators and stretched. The twenty-seven-year-old research officer was wearing faded Wrangler blue jeans and, worn one over the other, two long-sleeved pullovers. He had enormous eyes, thinning black hair, and a dimple in his chin. Nine color photographs of koala bears were pinned to the wall. One carried a cricket bat; another wore boxing gloves. A third sat on a director's chair. There was a passing resemblance between the prototype of the teddy bear and the earnest young Australian scientist.

While Cohen's team in New York struggled to master the microinjection technique, Sakkis had mastered it. It was hard to catch a single sperm, Sakkis said; they were sticky. It was even harder not to crush one. "We go into the sperm droplet, pick up the sperm, and inject it," he said. "You actually keep a buffer zone between the egg and the needle. You make a kind of furrow." On this day in December 1989, he had been working with mice. For almost four years, he had waited to perform the same procedure on human sperm and eggs. In Melbourne, the law wouldn't let him. Sakkis had taken over the experiment from other less-patient scientists. Now he was anxious to make up for lost time.

Three months earlier, the Centre had secured legal permission to perform the experiment on human embryos. Since then, Sakkis and his colleague, Orly Lacham, had inserted sperm—no more than three or four individual cells at a time—into eggs for 52 couples unable to conceive due to severe male infertility. About one-third of the eggs subsequently fertilized. So far, at least three women had become pregnant. They crossed their fingers in the hopes that the pregnancies would last, that the children they had conceived would be normal.

Sakkis and Lacham had missed their chance to achieve the world's first pregnancy from the technique. A clinic in Singapore had earned that medical honor. A few months later, a clinic in Sydney announced that it, too, had made a woman pregnant using sperm microinjection. Then another woman in Singapore became pregnant. Now there were rumors of a pregnancy in Italy. By the time Centre researchers finally achieved pregnancies with the microinjection technique they had pioneered, it was old news.

So the Monash Centre, which had won the race in the laboratory, found itself bringing up the rear—paralyzed by an intractable political debate over a scientist's right to intervene in the earliest beginnings of human life.

In Melbourne, capital city of the Australian state of Victoria, the sun was strong enough to peel paint. Palm trees spread their fronds amid the city's tarnished domes and Gothic spires. The city's distinctive green-and-yellow trolleys rumbled along broad avenues lined with lush hothouse greenery. It was a city of tropical climate and temperate habits, of provincial prudery and tabloid sensationalism. Shrieking kookaburra birds strutted on the sidewalks. At the southern tip of Port Phillip Bay, penguins burrowed among the roots of cypress trees. Koala bears hung like heavy fruit in the eucalyptus groves, the hot wind through the branches as aromatic as breath flavored by an old-fashioned cough drop.

Nowhere in the world had the subject of reproduction outside the human body been so publicly and thoroughly debated than in Victoria. Nowhere was the art of human embryology so advanced. By 1990, one in every 200 babies born in Australia was conceived artificially. Ironically, the slow-moving koalas—international symbols of The Land Down Under—had been struck by a plague of venereal disease so severe that it rendered almost every koala bear in the wild infertile and reduced the number of newborn bears to only ten a year. The Infertility Medical Centre at Epworth Hospital in Melbourne was one of the world's largest conception clinics. The Monash Centre led by Trounson was the world's largest single research establishment devoted to the basic investigation of human reproduction. Nowhere was such research so strictly controlled by law.

"We are talking about the development in a laboratory of the beginnings of human life—something that was never done before our time," said Louis Waller, a law professor who ran the committee that regulated embryo research. "It's something that keeps pulling us up short, just like the splitting of the atom did. Where do we strike the balance?"

More than any other single scientist, Alan Trounson invented the clinical practice of laboratory conception. To British pioneers Edwards and Steptoe belonged the honor of being first to conceive a test-tube baby. If the English proved it possible, however, the Australians made it practical. As it was practiced in hundreds of infertility clinics throughout the world, laboratory conception relied almost completely on the techniques developed by Trounson and his fellow Australians. Where the English pioneers were secretive, the Australians shared their work freely.

It was Trounson—working with his medical partners in Melbourne, Dr. Carl Wood and Dr. John Leeton—who perfected the use of fertility drugs that enabled doctors to cultivate dozens of human eggs at once. He also perfected the transfer of multiple human embryos. In 1984, he was the first to achieve human pregnancies with frozen embryos. The mother of the first boy nicknamed the child "Frostie." Trounson was the first to make women pregnant with donated human embryos.

In the end, one too many miracles came out of his laboratory. "Every day, frontiers were being pushed back again and again," said Dr. Ian Johnston, who was responsible for Australia's first test-tube baby. "It scared everyone. Melbourne suffered future shock." The local press turned against Trounson and his colleagues. Local religious leaders voiced misgivings about what they saw as medical meddling in the beginnings of life. Feminists were outraged by what they saw as exploitation of female research subjects. The government stepped in.

"I was just basically translating all of the things that I had developed and had learned in the animal industries. Super-ovulation. Freezing. Embryo transfer. With some modification, they fit the human beautifully," Trounson said.

The plainspoken Australian scientist looked as if he would be more comfortable manhandling stumps and fence posts than manipulating human embryos. Trounson, forty-four, was all chest and shoulders; his bushy brown hair was windblown. He seemed to own only one tie and one blue blazer, which he wore over acid-washed jeans and battered brogans in absentminded deference to the government ministers he outraged so regularly.

As a fresh-faced graduate student in veterinary science, Trounson mastered his craft in the arid Australian savannah of New South Wales. Instead of an embryo laboratory, he and his doctoral adviser tended a herd of 60,000 sheep on a 30,000-acre research station. Every day Trounson would kill a couple of sheep and dissect them to see what was going on inside.

"So sheep were like mice. We could do experiments involving a hundred animals at a time, herd them in and take all the eggs and embryos out of them."

For six years, he studied fertilization and embryo development in the sheep, using embryo transfer techniques. He traveled to England for two more years of advanced work at Cambridge University. But not until Wood brought him home to Melbourne in 1975, on a Ford Foundation grant for research into new forms of contraception, did Trounson see his first human embryo.

"I'd never even heard of infertility," Trounson said.

By the beginning of 1985, Trounson's team at the Monash Centre had perfected the laboratory skills needed to inject a single sperm cell into an egg. The scientists worried about the physical risk of replacing embryos from altered human eggs in a woman, without first assessing the risk of genetic damage.

"In the human, we will eventually be dealing with a child, so we'd better be correct," Trounson said.

They wanted to create several dozen human embryos with

the technique and then destroy them to analyze the chromosomes and genes. They had to be certain there were no subtle abnormalities that could result in a child with a birth defect. Under Victorian law, they would need the permission of Louis Waller's regulations committee.

Trounson wrote Waller to alert him privately to the pending research proposal. By 1988, the nine-member committee had debated the question at six major meetings. The committee was not blindly opposed to embryo research, but it believed it was wrong to destroy a human embryo deliberately for the sake of an experiment. They were determined that scientists should not be allowed to create life for the purpose of destroying it. They deliberated at such length that some of the scientists who were originally involved in the microinjection project accepted jobs in other countries. The committee finally decided that, before the experiment could proceed, the law itself had to be amended.

Orly Lacham, twenty-eight, was a visiting embryologist from Israel. She usually sat next to Sakkis in the Centre's embryo lab. Strong-willed, strong-jawed, red-haired, she fumed while the committee debated, argued, considered, tabled, and reconsidered. One day in July 1988, Lacham quietly gathered her notes, packed a suitcase, and caught a plane to Sydney. There, she conducted the embryo experiments the authorities in Victoria had forbidden.

She said it was an act of scientific responsibility; they would not risk the chance that an altered embryo would result in a deformed child. Lacham had to kill the embryos to see if they were normal. To those who believed that human life began at conception, they were a human sacrifice. But there was no shortage of clinics willing to transfer the altered embryos directly into a woman without taking any extra precautions. These clinics trusted the womb to bury their mistakes.

"We had to go out to Sydney in order to do this research, so we could say to the world: Okay, this technique is good enough to use in human beings," Lacham said. "I remember those days just before I went off to Sydney, when we were waiting for the committee here in Victoria to say yes. Every day we were waiting. They'd say: Maybe yes, maybe no, maybe yes, maybe no. We'd sit and sit and wait and wait. As a scientist I want to do things, I wanted to conduct these experiments that I knew I was not going to be allowed to conduct," she said.

In Sydney, she quickly discovered that the embryos were normal. She also taught embryologists at the Sydney IVF clinic how to use microsurgery to inject single sperm into eggs. Earlier, Trounson's team had shared its technique with embryologists at the Singapore IVF clinic. When each clinic announced its pregnancies, they made no mention of the Monash Centre's role. Lacham and Sakkis took a certain pride in them, anyway.

Quite clearly, they looked on their defiance of the rules as an act of self-restraint. "Even though we were one of the first groups that had the technique, we still didn't go ahead blindly and try to get the first pregnancy. We actually tried to verify the technique to see if it was safe to use first," Sakkis said. "We were the only group in the world to do that."

Public-health officials in Victoria were furious that Trounson had sidestepped their authority. There was not very much they could do about it except grant permission to perform the experiment locally—permission they had withheld for almost three years.

The Centre researchers had voluntarily submitted to regulation. Theirs was a show of goodwill, and political common sense. But the interminable debates exhausted their patience. "We are no longer number one. We should have fought more vigorously. We are being bullied," said Centre associate director Ismail Koler. Trounson, however, was used to the political minuet. He had been contending with periodic research moratoriums since 1982. He had been threatening to resign since 1983.

Within a few months, however, the government again would halt the Centre's experiments. This time, Trounson and his colleagues sought permission to dissect 100 two-day-old human embryos. Their aim was to test an embryo biopsy technique designed to detect gross chromosomal abnormalities. Instead, they touched off another political furor.

Again they found themselves testing the limits of acceptable research on the earliest stages of human life. Once more, government officials were alarmed over the destruction of human embryos. This time, however, Waller's committee quickly approved the experiment, but the state health minister overruled them. She suspended the work, banning any experiments with human embryos until "all the issues, legal and scientific, have been fully debated."

After almost a decade of uninterrupted public discussion about laboratory conception, the Monash scientists wondered what there was left to debate. The moratorium halted experiments on embryos more than 22 hours old—the moment when, at least in Victoria, life officially began. It suspended tests to determine sex and genetic disorders, but not routine clinical IVF work or the sperm experiments. Two Waller committee members, calling the minister's interference "abhorrent," resigned in protest. The moratorium was meant to last only a month or two, but it stretched on for more than a year with no end in sight. The lead scientist quit and moved to England. Others soon followed.

"In the case of the sperm microinjection experiment, I lost every one of the seven or eight people on the original research team. By the time we really were allowed to do it, we had to retrain everybody," Trounson said. "In the embryo biopsy experiment that's now under moratorium, nobody's left in the group, not a single scientist. So we will have to train someone else again. In the meantime, progress has gone on in other parts of the world where they've gone further and faster."

Trounson stared ruefully at the blisters that reddened his palms after a weekend's work on his 65-acre farm. After a decade as the world's most influential clinical embryologist, he talked like a man who might, any minute, quit to raise sheep in the country. The Australian researchers who had done so much to make laboratory conception practical were blocked from further improving it. As a consequence, infertile men and women would have to live with the clinical flaws that kept success rates so low.

"Our direct involvement in human reproductive medicine has declined and will continue to decline. We will contribute a relatively small component of the worldwide research,"

Trounson said, "unless we go to another place and do the research there."

In the meantime, Sakkis and Lacham proceeded with their sperm microinjection experiment undisturbed. Hospital space was so limited that they had to set up their microsurgery tools in a building far from the operating room and the embryo lab. They carried the embryos from one building to the next, up and down stairs, in and out of elevators. "We haven't had an accident yet," said embryologist Theresa Brady.

She pointed to a large gray vat in the corner. It contained more than 400 frozen embryos. Some of them had been in cold storage for seven years.

"The laws in Victoria are strange," Brady said. "Couples are allowed to donate embryos for research, but you are not allowed to conduct any research. So they sit there."

In Atlanta and New York, Jacques Cohen's "PZD" microsurgery was working so well that he was even more convinced that the tiny holes he made in human eggs and embryos could revolutionize the practice of laboratory conception. By the spring of 1990, Cohen and his colleagues at Reproductive Biology Associates and Cornell had surgically altered eggs for 212 couples. Forty-two became pregnant. Almost 20 babies had been born. All were healthy. The rate at which his altered embryos implanted in the womb was consistently twice the national average.

Despite the clinical success, Jacques Cohen could tell that many of his altered embryos were abnormal just by looking at them under the microscope. A newly fertilized egg normally displayed two small shadowy spheres called pronuclei that held the key to the fate of the newly created organism. Each contained a tiny packet of genes: one from the mother's egg, the other from the father's sperm. In the surgically altered embryos, Cohen often saw three.

If transplanted to a woman, such an abnormal embryo often aborted within a few weeks. But if it survived, the resulting child would, at best, be mentally retarded and die within a few days of birth. The risk was so great that embryologists routinely discarded all abnormal embryos. It was great enough that many doctors questioned the wisdom of trying to fertilize any human egg more than once. It was a fear that plagued them from the earliest days of laboratory conception. While they awaited the birth of the first test-tube baby, Steptoe and Edwards kept secret the fact that one of the embryos they had created and implanted in their first set of experimental pregnancies was genetically abnormal. The woman carrying it miscarried. Tests revealed the fetus had an extra set of chromosomes. Subsequently, they made all the women participating in the experiment agree in advance to an abortion should tests reveal that the embryos had developed into an abnormal fetus.

Cohen and other researchers sought to repair those defective embryos. They were scientists struggling to fix the mistakes their science had created. They surgically removed the extra pronucleus by sucking it up with a microscopic syringe. In published papers, they called the microsurgical repair "enucleation." In the lab, Cohen called it "slurping."

"A slurp is a traumatic thing," Henry Malter said. It was also dangerous. There was no reliable way to tell whether the right bundle of chromosomes had been removed.

If the scientists slurped the wrong one or left any fragments of the extra male pronucleus, they only added to the embryo's abnormalities. If they cut out the female pronucleus by mistake, they could create a lethal condition in which the embryo never stopped growing inside the womb. "It's like *Alien*— something which takes over your body," said Cohen. "It is one of the most spooky things in reproduction."

Surprisingly, many embryos survived even this surgical shock to their system. At a time when the embryo consisted of only a few cells, it could lose more than half of them and still grow into a normal child. In France and Spain, women had been made pregnant with the remnants of what had originally been four-cell embryos.

"We had one baby from a half-embryo in Atlanta," Cohen said. "The baby already is fine. The mother was never told that this was half an embryo."

The slurp—and other microsurgical procedures like it— transformed laboratory conception from a treatment for infertility into a tool for genetic testing. The slurp opened the door to genetic analysis of embryos for sex, disease, or any other characteristic for which geneticists could devise a DNA probe. The test results could be available within hours. The entire procedure need take no more than a day. Defective embryos would be thrown away or saved for research. Genetically "clean" embryos could be implanted just as in any other IVF embryo transfer.

As soon as he knew he was removing the correct pronucleus, Cohen would offer the altered embryos to human patients. "It will be the first genetic repair in the human being—the repair of polyspermic embryos," he said. "It will be important for ethicists to consider this. We will be taking a highly abnormal embryo containing two sperm and making it a normal embryo."

5

The Mouse Is a Tomato

The procedures manual for laboratory conception told one creation story. Computer printouts of the human genetic sequence told another.

For those who could read it, the human sequence was a diary of Genesis, the genetic record of a family so large it encompassed all organic life. In it, molecular biologists traced the tale of an aboriginal Eve and the ascent of man. They discovered a brotherhood of fruit flies, mice, and men—a kinship linking all life in test-tube Earth.

In its unabridged version, this human volume contained a single repetitive sentence billions of letters long—a terse chemical description that would fill 200 books the thickness of the Manhattan telephone directory. This was the construction kit for the molecular machine called humankind—a word made flesh. As researchers identified and analyzed the genes responsible for growth and development, they deciphered the enduring mystery of how a human being develops from a single fertilized cell. Parents weren't the only ones who wondered how a baby could come from something so small.

The human genome, as molecular biologists termed the genetic text for assembling a man or a woman, contained as many separate chemical base pairs of DNA as there were persons living in the world. No one knew how many genes it contained, perhaps as many as 100,000. The double strands of DNA in each cell made a twisted thread more than five feet long and just 50 trillionths of an inch wide. It was different for every human being but virtually identical inside each of the body's 10 trillion cells.

It linked all living organisms. Only two million base pairs separated brother and sister. Between a human being and a chimpanzee, the difference was about 50 million more base pairs; between mice and men, 100 million more base pairs; between humanity and a leaf of spinach, a difference of two billion base pairs.

Biologists who studied these genes talked prophetically of predictive medicine and promised they would forever alter the way doctors treated disease. The growing awareness of the genetic causes of illness had a subtle side effect—the patient became the disease. A defective gene was an integral part of the unique genome that produced each child—as much a bequest of the parents who conceived him or her as blue eyes or black skin.

There are more than 3,000 known genetic diseases. In the United States alone, inherited illnesses hospitalized 1.2 million people a year, at a cost of $2.35 billion. They killed one of every five newborns, caused half the nation's miscarriages, and were responsible for eight of every 10 cases of mental retardation. In all, 12 million Americans were afflicted by genetic disorders, but scientists believed that every individual alive carried a handful of genes that could result in a child with a birth defect or inherited disorder.

Conventional prenatal diagnosis posed an agonizing choice for parents. If a serious inherited defect was found in a fetus, a doctor often could treat the disease only by eliminating the patient. Parents weighed the moral cost of abortion against the moral cost of giving birth to an affected child. They wanted a healthy child, and they wanted a clear conscience. With conventional prenatal diagnostic tests, couples endured weeks of uncertainty awaiting test results. Many couples, faced with the prospect of a therapeutic abortion, were afraid to acknowledge the developing fetus until it received a clean bill of genetic health. Others refused to have anything to do with prenatal tests.

Researchers were learning to diagnose disease genes in single sperm, eggs, and embryos. With a single cell removed from a human embryo within hours of conception, scientists could determine its sex and, with increasing certainty, also predict its susceptibility to many inherited diseases—both without affecting its ability to develop into a normal baby. Laboratory conception, developed to treat infertility, was being turned to broader medical applications. And what scientists couldn't cure, they could eliminate.

Accurate diagnosis of an embryo would enable women to avoid bearing children with an inherited disease by relying on laboratory conception. Technicians could inspect the embryos and guarantee that none carrying the lethal gene would be allowed to survive by simply leaving them in their laboratory dish. With abortion facing an uncertain future in many parts of the United States, the additional medical inconvenience and uncertainty of laboratory conception could become a legal necessity for couples seeking to avoid offspring with a genetic disease.

For those scientists involved in laboratory conception, genetic testing was a natural outgrowth of the attitude they brought to their infertility work: They could not cure infertility, but they could circumvent the medical conditions barring conception to make babies. They could not cure any of the genetic diseases, but, with genetic diagnosis of embryos, they could create children that did not inherit them. Couples in the United States commonly used donor sperm to avoid passing an inherited disease from the husband. Couples could conceive with donor eggs to avoid passing on a hereditary disease from the wife.

For Dr. Gary Hodgen, scientific director at the Jones Institute, the marriage of human genetics and assisted reproduction technology was a natural union. "The whole reproductive process is for a single purpose—to pass DNA from one generation to the next. Not a single other thing is important. Anything that does not meet the purpose of passing DNA between generations is not going to be supported by evolution and shouldn't be supported by the scientific process. The behavior that leads to the romance, the copulation that leads to the fertilization, the implantation, the placenta, the delivery, the breast-feeding—everything is conjured directly by nature to see that DNA is transferred. That alone is the bull's-eye.

"The ultimate importance of IVF is not the treatment of infertility," Dr. Hodgen said, "but the capacity to prevent the human suffering that occurs as a result of genetically inherited diseases. That suffering not only involves the individual with the inherited disease. It also is the suffering of the siblings, the parents, the grandparents, the larger family, and, in fact, all of us."

For embryologists, human life was a matter of cells; for geneticists, it was a question of molecules. They worked to the same fundamental purpose: to understand and control how human beings transformed themselves into succeeding generations. Doctors counseled infertile couples; embryologists manipulated the sperm and eggs they produced; molecular biologists analyzed the genes and chromosomes inside them. In the embryo labs, technicians prodded human reproductive material with glass pipettes and microneedles. Molecular biologists used enzymes and proteins to chemically cut and splice the genes of choice.

Scientists painfully mastered the genetic language of life. They learned its grammar, verb structure, and punctuation. They used the knowledge to edit sentences into new life-forms—bacteria that secreted human insulin, crops that produced their own pesticide and weed killer, mice and sheep that gave human heart medicine in their milk. Some of the life-forms were technical stunts: tobacco plants that glow in the dark. Some of them were unsettling: pink petunias containing genes for human fertility hormones. Some of them, such as the genetically engineered pigs, were crippled.

On paper, the DNA formula was life stripped of its living things. The banded maps of chromosomes were human bar codes. Some researchers worried that they had become so enthralled by the mysteries of the genetic code they had forgotten that any of it involved living cells. Viewed from inside the genetic labyrinth, the cells all seemed so interchangeable. "To a geneticist, a tomato is virtually identical to a mouse," said Eric Lander at the Whitehead Institute of Biomedical Research in Cambridge, Massachusetts. What they could do with a tomato, they often could do with a laboratory mouse—and one day soon they hoped to be able to duplicate with the human genetic structure.

Geneticists and molecular biologists had already transformed the understanding of conception. They discovered that men and women were not necessarily equal partners in the genetic merger that took place inside a fertilized human egg. A gene inherited from one parent could behave differently from the same gene passed on by the other parent. This "genetic imprinting" meant that some genes would work in an embryo only if they were inherited from a man; others would function only if they were passed on by a woman. In some species, an egg could be prodded into development without fertilization, but not among mammals. Many biologists believed imprinting was the reason chromosomes from a male—and not just any chromosome—were required for normal development in a mammalian egg.

They were redrawing the human family tree. They discovered an entirely separate pattern of inheritance that, contained within the ancient vestigial bacteria called mitochondria inside the human egg, was passed on exclusively through women. The mitochondria, free-floating bodies inside every living cell that provided much of the cell's energy, were a remnant of a time when single-cell organisms first joined together in symbiosis to make more complex life-forms. Each new human generation received an almost exact copy of the mitochondrial genes of their maternal forebears, altered only by the occasional genetic mutation. Scientists at Emory University and the University of California—molecular anthropologists who analyzed mitochondria instead of hominid fossils—argued that all humans living today were descended from one common ancestor, a woman who lived more than 200,000 years ago. This ancestral Eve roamed the plains of Africa or perhaps Asia. They traced nearly all American Indians, including the Mayans, Incas, and many others spread throughout North, Central, and South America, to four women who walked across what is now the Bering Strait more than 15,000 years ago in a single small band. In the mutations of those genes, they uncovered a previously unsuspected group of inherited diseases that sapped each cell's ability to produce energy, causing muscle disorders and blindness.

While clinical embryologists funded their work with patients' gifts and private grants, molecular biologists and medical geneticists thrived on lavish federal support, totaling more than $200 million a year. After four years of debate, the federal government in 1990 launched its most ambitious human biology project yet: a $3 billion, 15-year effort to locate, map, and analyze every one of the 100,000 human genes that shape a human being from embryo to adult. Project officials were so concerned about the possible general backlash stemming from human genome research that they pledged three percent of the project's estimated budget—about $90 million—for an unprecedented effort to examine the ethical, legal, and social implications of decoding all human genes.

The increasing knowledge of genes accelerated the commercialization of the human body. Doctors and patients faced off in court over who owned an individual's cells and the genes they contained. Researchers argued over whether the human genome itself should be subject to copyright. A few profitable fragments of it had been patented by pharmaceutical companies. Genetic identity, like public reputation, had become property. "I certainly consider my genetic sequence my property," said Dr. Charles Cantor, head of the human genome program at Lawrence Berkeley Laboratory at the University of California.

"Powerful new technologies do not just change what we can do," said public-health law analyst George J. Annas at Boston University. "They also change the way we think—especially about ourselves." The human genome project promised to alter the ideas of what it meant to be human as completely as Columbus's voyage to America changed the shape of the world. The breakthroughs in genetics already had turned the biological barriers between species into a revolving door. It made a child an assembly of molecules. "We will have a human being made up of small parts, all of them interchangeable," Annas said.

It altered ideas of ownership. The U.S. courts ruled that biologists could patent their new life-forms, even if their creations utilized human genes. In 1988, a mouse prone to human breast cancer, genetically engineered at Harvard University, became the world's first patented animal. U.S. Patent number 4,736,866 was assigned to the President and Fellows of Harvard College, covering virtually any species of "transgenic nonhuman mammal all of whose germ cells and somatic cells contain a recombinant activated oncogene sequence introduced into said mammal or an ancestor of said mammal, at an embryonic stage."

E.I. Du Pont de Nemours & Co., which licensed the genetically engineered mouse from Harvard, marketed it as the "OncoMouse" and sold it at $50 each—10 times the price of stock laboratory mice. Company officials said they expected to sell up to $25 million worth of man-made mice every year.

It was not the high price that raised eyebrows, however; it was Du Pont's unusual marketing strategy. The multinational chemical company would not actually sell its living product to anyone. It would only license the mice—not unlike computer software. The company retained the legal title. The arrangement, called bailment, permitted the company to retain an interest in the mouse and all of its descendants. People wondered at the precedent that had been set. In the same year, the European Patent Office had turned down Harvard's application on the grounds that higher life-forms cannot be patented. Many countries had made it a crime to combine human and animal gametes at the cellular level of sperm and egg. In the case of the OncoMouse and a flood of other such living products, scientists were offered commercial protection when, at the molecular level, they combined human and animal genes.

Mastery of the genetic code gave the human embryo a new identity. The early human embryo, smaller than the period at the end of a sentence, was the repository of a uniquely individual genetic sequence. In some courtrooms, it had become father to the man. "The two-cell embryo is genetically the process of transmitting information from the parents to the child in the smallest possible language," testified Dr. Jerome Lejeune, a noted French geneticist, in a Tennessee divorce dispute over frozen embryos. Life begins at conception, he said. The embryos were early human beings. "The information inside this cell has all the tricks of the trade—how to live," he said. "As soon as he is conceived, a man is a man."

Opposing attorney Charles Clifford pondered Lejeune's testimony about human beginnings, and, when it was his turn to question the scientist, he held up a white hen's egg. "Do you know what this is?" he asked Lejeune.

"An egg," the Frenchman responded.

"Good," said Clifford. "I thought you were going to tell me it was an early chicken."

For many, the most important knowledge to be gleaned from the genome revealed the role played by heredity in human disease. Even a flaw in a single gene could be fatal. Since 1950, when scientists weren't even sure how many chromosomes a human cell contained, biologists had identified some 3,000 diseases caused by microscopic defects in the genome. Some were so rare that they affected no more than 40 people worldwide. One blinded the 100,000 Americans who inherited it. One in every 12 American blacks carried a gene for sickle-cell anemia. One in every 30 Ashkenazi Jews carried a gene for Tay-Sachs disease. One in every 25 Caucasians carried a gene for cystic fibrosis. Researchers also found suggestive genetic links to more complex behavior-related conditions like heart disease, alcoholism, and mental illness. One gene, inherited by more than one-third of the population, could triple the risk of a heart attack. Others made the people who carried them more susceptible to cancer. Scientists detected a genetic factor that influenced how quickly a person became ill after being infected by the AIDS virus.

Researchers promised to generate thousands of inexpensive genetic tests. Each new test turned a human gene into a medical prophecy—sometimes as chillingly clear as a courtroom death sentence; at other times as obscure as the predictions of the Delphic oracle.

It was, most intimately, a question of family.

Geneticists gleaned their earliest and strongest evidence of disease genes from genealogies. In the family trees of North Georgia mountain clans, among the isolated communities of the Old Order Amish in Lancaster County, Pennsylvania, and among the extended families along Lake Maracaibo in Venezuela, researchers isolated the patterns of inheritance. One family was prone to suicide and depression; another had an unusually high incidence of muscular dystrophy; a third passed Huntington's chorea from generation to generation. Researchers discovered genetic markers that, like red flags, revealed the presence of each disease gene well before any symptoms of the disease appeared. They could follow it through the generations even when the gene itself was unknown. "The location of the gene is embedded in the pattern of inheritance," said Ray White, a senior researcher at the Howard Hughes Medical Institute in Utah.

Narrowing the search was tedious and expensive. To locate the gene responsible for cystic fibrosis, for example, researchers spent about $120 million. The medical and commercial incentives were enormous. Cystic fibrosis was potentially the most lethal gene in North America. A comprehensive genetic test would cost about $200. Up to three million people a year could be considered candidates for testing. Within a year of isolating the cystic fibrosis gene, scientists were able to cure cells in a test tube that contained it by altering their genetic structure.

In the archives of the Mormon Church, researchers sought evidence of family links to chronic diseases like high blood pressure, coronary heart disease, and cancer. For a century, the LDS Genealogical Library in Salt Lake City had been building the most extensive family records in existence—more than 88 million names, 25 million parish records, 8 million family trees, and thousands of immigrant manifests, military personnel records, census results, court records, and trust deeds from all over the world. They were so important to the Church that duplicates were secreted in the granite heart of the Rocky Mountains—secure from fire, flood, and nuclear war. To population geneticists they were equally precious. At the University of Utah, they linked the Mormon records to state birth certificates, state cancer registries, and hospital files, and created a unique medical genealogy encompassing 1.3 million people. They turned Utah itself into a living genetics laboratory.

The nagging questions of heredity were as old as family and the idea of the "bad seed." Molecular biology, coupled with laboratory conception and computerized medical records, lent them an added urgency.

Such genetic records contained a special knowledge that affected more than just the individual whose name was on the file. It affected entire families who shared common ancestors. It was knowledge that was easily misunderstood and readily misused. In the United States, compulsory genetic screening for sickle-cell anemia during the 1970s became a tool of discrimination to deny blacks jobs, insurance coverage, and military training. Earlier ideas of genetic purity spawned laws regulating marriage, enforced sterilization, immigration restrictions, and permanent confinement of genetic "misfits." At least 30 states had laws dealing with "hereditary defectives" well before Nazi Germany passed its first hereditary health law. In the Soviet Union, misguided notions of genetics were enforced by the secret police.

Half a century later, Fortune 500 firms used genetic tests as part of routine executive physicals. Congressional experts determined that at least 22 U.S. companies were developing commercial genetic tests for a $200-million-a-year testing business. A dozen companies used them to screen employees. Market forecasts suggested that by the mid-1990s, 30 million genetic tests would be given annually to diagnose the earliest signs of cancer, heart disease, and hereditary disorders. Virginia and 11 other states kept data banks of genetic material from convicted criminals. The Federal Bureau of Investigation, which already conducted DNA tests for police departments around the country, studied how to link the state DNA banks in a national network. As concern over each individual's genetic family tree increased, the nation's largest private genetic-testing laboratory opened a commercial DNA storage center that offered to "bank" cells from every member of a family for a onetime deposit fee of $150. No matter how many genetic tests were developed in the future, the raw human material would always be available for analysis and comparison with the genes their descendants had inherited. "By storing specimens of DNA from family members now, families may be assured that their children and grandchildren will not be excluded from testing in the future," explained a spokesman for the Vivigen Genetic Repository in Santa Fe, New Mexico.

To contain spiraling medical-care costs, would the insurance companies use genetic tests to deny medical benefits to a couple who bore an affected child? All 50 states required newborn infants to be tested for one or more inherited diseases. The Medical Information Bureau, which served 700 insurance companies, maintained detailed health records on 11 million people. Passive carriers of sickle-cell anemia and Gaucher disease had been denied insurance even though they displayed no symptoms of the disease for which they carried a single gene. People who inherited rare hereditary disorders such as Charcot-Marie-Tooth muscular atrophy and a neurodegenerative disorder called Friedrich's Ataxia had also been denied coverage. In 1990, to ensure that the right to privacy extended to an individual's genetic makeup, U.S. Representative John Conyers, D-Mich., introduced the first federal legislation of its kind to explicitly prohibit discrimination based on a genetic diagnosis or screening test. Twenty countries were considering similar legislation.

Would employers screen employees to keep insurance premiums down? Some chemical companies already had, refusing to hire minorities who showed an inborn sensitivity to manufacturing compounds. In 1989, 20 U.S. companies said they performed genetic tests on employees. How would doctors counsel a family in which they could diagnose, but could not cure or treat, a fatal hereditary disease? Would doctors be sued if they did not offer a prenatal genetic test? Some physicians had already been forced to defend their actions in court, sued by angry parents for the "wrongful life" of an afflicted child. Did a woman have a right to bear an afflicted child that society would have to bear the costs of raising? Was *she* a criminal?

Each new probe and the gene that it identified posed its

own unique social riddles. There was no federal regulation of prenatal testing, nor of commercial or clinical genetics. There was, for example, no formal public consideration of DNA fingerprinting before commercial firms aggressively marketed the technique as the scientific answer to a prosecutor's prayer. Only later, after police had used it in more than 2,000 criminal investigations, was its infallibility challenged—when, in court, defense attorneys uncovered troubling flaws in laboratory quality controls. As medical clinical services, the cascade of new genetic tests bypassed regulations aimed at research. Their clinical use was considered a matter of professional judgment. That judgment was, in turn, shaped by commercial pressures, malpractice premiums, and the fear of litigation. The American Medical Association estimated the annual cost of "defensive medicine" at about $15.5 billion. That was the price of the extra procedures and tests ordered by doctors simply to lessen the risk of a malpractice lawsuit. The use of the newest DNA tests would be a matter of conscience and the threat of procreative product liability.

In 1927, the U.S. Supreme Court sanctioned the involuntary sterilization of the mentally retarded because, just as the state had the right to expect its citizens to lay down their lives in wartime for the common good, it had an equal right to prevent "defectives" from having children. Sixty years later, the congressional Office of Technology Assessment advised Congress that genetic testing could be a useful tool for cost-containment. "Human mating that proceeds without the use of genetic data about the risks of transmitting diseases will produce greater mortality and medical costs than if carriers of potentially deleterious genes are alerted to their status and encouraged to mate with noncarriers or to use artificial insemination or other reproductive strategies." Separated by three generations, the words echoed a public-health ethic in which the abnormal was seen as disposable. The budget imperatives of the medical marketplace reinforced ideas of genetic purity.

Amniocentesis could detect fetal abnormalities after about 15 weeks of gestation, with test results usually not ready until a fetus had reached about 22 weeks. Chorionic villus sampling could detect them by the eighth week of a pregnancy. If the test revealed evidence of an inherited disease, there usually was no cure—only the possibility of an abortion.

Once doctors could screen human embryos, however, parents could theoretically know from the start that their child would have healthy genes. Already, a few researchers were taking prenatal diagnosis into the instant of conception itself.

"I fear the aspiration for the perfect child," said James M. Gustafson, a leading authority on religion, ethics, and law at Emory University, "and the misconceptions that might be forthcoming."

There was something about the painting on the gallery wall that made Yuri Verlinsky think about human eggs. Miró was never his favorite artist. But in 1989 on an idle April afternoon in Tel Aviv, the Spanish painter's dreamy geometry triggered an idea.

Verlinsky's group at the Reproductive Genetics Institute in Chicago specialized in reproductive genetics. He had helped pioneer chorionic villus sampling in the United States. Every year, his group conducted genetic tests on fetuses in 2,000 pregnant women. "The next step was to analyze the embryo before we put it back in a woman," Verlinsky said. The painting suggested a way.

Miró had painted two enormous disks. To Verlinsky's eye, they looked like human eggs. To one clung a small black sphere. The second disk was by itself, as if the small sphere had been excised. "Ah," the Russian-émigré geneticist said to himself, "there is one egg with a polar body and another egg without one." The polar body is a tiny packet of chromosomes present in all human eggs that is normally sloughed off before the egg is fertilized. If Verlinsky could surgically extract a polar body from a human egg, he could perform prenatal diagnostic tests by analyzing the genetic material it contained. He would be able to diagnose some hereditary disorders passed on by the mother before the egg and sperm actually joined.

Later that day at the King David Hotel, he sought out Jacques Cohen. Was it possible to surgically extract that bit of tissue safely, without damaging the egg? Absolutely, Cohen replied. When he slit the zona membrane around the egg for his PZD procedure, he often destroyed that polar body with no apparent ill effects. The resulting embryos developed normally, Cohen said. Verlinsky was elated. He scribbled his idea on a business card and took it back to his laboratory.

Using the microsurgery developed by Cohen to slurp embryos, Verlinsky's team at the Illinois Masonic Medical Center extracted the polar body. During the natural development of the egg, the woman's complete set of genes was divided equally between the mature egg and the polar body. When they amplified and analyzed the genetic material the polar body contained, the scientists could deduce whether the egg itself was healthy. In some cases, they were able to diagnose common disorders such as cystic fibrosis and a common form of mental retardation inherited by men called fragile-X syndrome. The resulting embryos went on to develop normally, apparently unharmed by the procedure. Verlinsky had quickly determined that the idea on the back on his business card worked. Almost as quickly, he was ready to create healthy embryos and transfer them into the wombs of human volunteers.

Five families volunteered for the experiment. But, because of the prevailing ban on research funding, no foundation would fund it; neither would the National Institutes of Health. Verlinsky and his colleague, Charles M. Strom, director of the center's medical genetics and DNA laboratory, decided to pay for the embryo diagnostic tests themselves. The patients paid for the fertility drugs they would need. The in vitro fertilization itself would otherwise be free to the volunteers. They were all on their own.

In a sense, they were lucky. The hospital did not receive any NIH funds, either, so the government could not block their embryo research by threatening to withdraw the hospital's grants. "We have no federal funding sources, so we don't have to conform to NIH guidelines. This probably could not be approved by NIH, anyway, given the current climate over there. Our hospital does not depend on NIH funds, so our institutional review board doesn't have to worry about being censored by the threat of having our NIH funds taken away," said Strom. "There's no academic center in this country that can really say the same. They would all be grievously injured if the NIH pulled their money out of it."

What they had instead of funding was the confidence of their ideas. Strom, a brawny Yale graduate with curly blond hair and thick, winglike eyebrows, rode around Chicago in a luxurious white Lincoln with the vanity license plate GENETICS. Verlinsky, an energetic Russian refugee with flushed cheeks and a wisp of a goatee, resembled an aging faun. He drove a chocolate-colored Porsche and dressed in double-breasted Italian suits. A native of Siberia, he had trained under a Soviet system in which it was not altogether unfortunate when the government ignored a scientist's work—especially if the scientist was studying heredity. Under Stalin, Soviet officials had embraced an especially political view of human genetics, which held that purely physical changes to an organism, such as a shortened tail in a mouse, could be inherited. Despite all the medical evidence to the contrary, Stalin embraced the idea and its orthodoxy was enforced by the secret police. Those who failed to toe the party's scientific line could be imprisoned or executed.

Verlinsky's procedure was elaborate. First, he analyzed the egg to sift out defects passed on by the mother. Those that were approved were fertilized. Then he performed a biopsy on the embryo to detect any defect inherited from the father. The team performed similar tests on eggs and embryos for couples with a history of cystic fibrosis, Tay-Sachs disease, hemophilia, a hereditary lung disease, and several inherited forms of mental retardation. Their first cystic fibrosis test was typical of the experiment: "We did the polar body biopsy. The polar body was normal so we knew the egg was abnormal. We fertilized the egg with the assumption it will be fertilized with a normal sperm. We did a biopsy on the embryo. It turned out the embryo would have had cystic fibrosis," Verlinsky said. The microsurgery took no more than five minutes. The test results were available in about five hours.

In the last stage of the experiment, the healthy embryos were transferred into the women. By the summer of 1990, however, only two women had become pregnant through the technique. Both women miscarried at 11 weeks. Verlinsky had yet to see a healthy baby born; nonetheless, a line had already formed at his laboratory door. Fifty couples called to volunteer. By September, a third woman was pregnant. Verlinsky kept the news to himself. He crossed his fingers.

"Some of these people had already used conventional pre-natal tests and terminated pregnancies," explained Strom. "These people are not opposed to pregnancy termination on religious or moral grounds, but they couldn't stand the nine weeks of not knowing and the nine weeks of being pregnant waiting for the prenatal test results. They said that was the worst two months of their life."

Prenatal diagnosis became pre-conception diagnosis. Even so sophisticated a prenatal technique was limited. It could only detect a handful of the inherited diseases that plagued human beings. Its safety was unproven. As expert an embryologist as IVF pioneer Robert Edwards was dubious; it involved too much guesswork. "I have my doubts about polar body analysis. Too much extrapolation. So much handling of the egg and em-bryos. That might have an adverse effect," he said. Better, he argued, to diagnose the embryo alone. Nonetheless, by screen-ing for faulty genes in unfertilized eggs, Verlinsky's team could allow thousands of women with a family history of genetic disorders to avoid giving birth to an afflicted child without having to undergo abortion. So far, they had only produced miscarriages.

"It is not additional risk," Verlinsky told his critics. "It is just risk."

Alan Handyside, stoop-shouldered, soft-spoken, with cool blue eyes and a narrow moustache trimmed to parallel his upper lip, was as anxious as any expectant father. Every year, 1,000 couples came to the outskirts of London for treatment at Hammersmith Hospital's infertility clinic, where he was chief embryologist. Hundreds became pregnant; hundreds more went home in disappointment. Children of two Arab royal families were conceived in its laboratory dishes. During 1989 and 1990, while Cohen perfected his microsurgery and

Verlinsky learned to diagnose hereditary flaws in human eggs, three pregnant women in particular had the English scientist's unwavering attention.

Each expectant mother was trying to avoid having a child with an inherited illness. One woman was a carrier of genes that caused a severe form of mental retardation. The other was a carrier for a childhood disease that caused progressive mental decay, blindness, and death. The third woman was a carrier for Duchenne's muscular dystrophy. But if Handyside had seen clearly into the chromosomes in the embryos he transferred into the women's wombs, the children they now carried would be born free of genetic disease.

Embryologists like Handyside were actively investigating ways to diagnose genetic diseases in human embryos. They sought to perfect the technique of testing the hereditary health of a living embryo without harming it. They took prenatal diagnosis into a moment when there was no fetus and, if a defective gene was detected, no necessity for therapeutic abortion. They used defective or spare, donated embryos to check the safety and practicality of their experimental tests before applying them in clinical volunteers.

Handyside and his colleagues at Hammersmith Hospital had used microsurgery and a genetic test to determine the sex of human embryos, so that doctors could discard any male embryos that might carry any one of 200 sex-linked inherited diseases. Many of them were so rare that their names could be found only in medical dictionaries. Some of them were among the most common hereditary diseases known, including muscular dystrophy, sickle-cell anemia, hemophilia and fragile-X syndrome. Together they affected millions worldwide. Several groups were testing human embryos for the mutation that caused cystic fibrosis. About eight million Americans—one out of every 20 who are of northern European origin—carry a gene for the disease.

"The first diagnosis we tackled wasn't really a diagnosis at all," Handyside said. "We tried to simply sex the embryos. We wanted to be as conservative as possible in the amount of material we take from the embryos. We found we can remove two cells from an eight-cell embryo without compromising the preimplantation embryo's development. The hole I make is relatively large."

By the spring of 1990, the research team had successfully impregnated two of the women with four female embryos whose sex was determined outside the womb. Both women were carrying twins. Handyside, who also was study director and senior lecturer at the Royal Postgraduate Medical School, said that ultrasound tests showed that the four fetuses were normal. The babies were due to be born four months after their arrival had been heralded in the science journal *Nature*. The third woman was in the early stages of a pregnancy with a single fetus.

"From the very first transfer, we had a biochemical pregnancy," Handyside said. "The great advantage here is being able to screen embryos without abortion."

In tests involving five women, four of 17 embryos screened prior to implantation, or 24 percent, had gone on to develop in the womb. That rate was twice the success rate for the regular transfer of test-tube embryos.

The English experiments grew out of a private meeting in 1986 underwritten by the Ciba Foundation. Twenty-five British scientists, including Robert Edwards, planned how they should develop "a form of prenatal diagnosis that would circumvent the need for selective abortion, at least while no means of corrective therapy is available." Three years later, the Hammersmith Hospital was offering embryo diagnosis to the first group of patients—years before most U.S. hospitals were willing to consider preliminary experiments with the technique.

English anti-abortion activists vehemently opposed the work. They argued that the embryo researchers were only developing a new form of prenatal euthanasia, not a true cure or treatment. When Parliament authorized human embryo experiments in 1990, Cardinal Basil Hume, the head of the Catholic Church in England and Wales, declared that England could no longer claim to be "a Christian society." Others less opposed to abortion itself grew uneasy about the proper limits on embryo research. For all the debate they generated, the embryo experiments had attracted only meager financial support. Although sanctioned by the British government, Handyside's work at Hammersmith was underwritten by a two-year, $71,000 grant from a private muscular dystrophy charity.

From Jacques Cohen's work, Handyside and his colleagues knew they could safely make a hole in an embryo. But would removing one or two cells affect later fetal development? Verlinsky's experiments in Chicago had all ended in miscarriages. "Nobody really knows what an embryo biopsy would do to a human," said Charles Strom. "Until Handyside's babies are born, we won't know for sure."

The embryo tests hinged on the ability of scientists to safely remove a cell from an embryo at a time when the entire organism consisted of only a few cells, and—even more important—the ability to analyze swiftly the genetic material it contained. The microsurgery developed by Cohen and other embryologists enabled technicians to siphon off safely a few cells for testing, but the genetic analysis itself was so expensive and time-consuming that most biologists dismissed the idea of ever conducting routine diagnostic tests on living embryos. The original tests required so many cells that to sample the embryo directly was to kill it.

In the United States and England, scientists had developed genetic "fingerprinting" using radioactive probes and lengthy laboratory tests. But genetic fingerprinting might involve millions of human cells. With that much genetic material to work with, there was little room for error. Researchers couldn't culture cells from an embryo fast enough for conventional genetic diagnosis. They often had only a single cell from which to work.

The breakthrough came in 1985 with a revolutionary technique invented by the Cetus Corporation in San Francisco. The company's genetic engineers harnessed the talents of an unusual bacteria discovered in a hot spring to accelerate DNA's natural ability to replicate itself. The new technique, called the polymerase chain reaction (PCR), could quickly and cheaply amplify the smallest samples of genetic material from a strand of hair, a drop of blood, or semen, into something large enough for a laboratory to analyze. It was so sensitive that it could detect and replicate the genetic sequence preserved in a fossil magnolia leaf that shaded the ancient relatives of elk and deer more than 17 million years ago. It enabled researchers to make hundreds of thousands of copies of the genes inside a single cell from an embryo in only hours. It was fast and inexpensive. In the three hours it took to complete 25 PCR cycles, a lab technician could amplify a cell 30-millionfold—fast enough so that genetic tests could be performed during a normal in vitro fertilization cycle.

"It's like a dream come true," said Alan Trounson.

As they began their first experiments with human volunteers, researchers were still concerned about the accuracy of the test itself. A false positive could mean that an embryo would be discarded unnecessarily. A false negative could mean that the woman might bear an affected child. Laboratory quality control was a matter of life and death. The nature of the early human embryo made the problem even harder to solve. In many species, the cells of the early embryo were uniform. But with human embryos, there was evidence suggesting that the cells often were different, like multicolored tiles in a mosaic. When the embryo consisted of only a few cells, all of them could be different. Tests on one cell would not necessarily reveal the characteristics of the entire human embryo.

"How in the hell do we pick out the right cell each time?" said Trounson. "Because if we're going to make a genetic diagnosis or a chromosomal diagnosis, it's got to be accurate."

The researchers faced an equally troubling problem with the PCR technology itself—it was almost too sensitive. When trying to amplify and analyze the genes from a single cell, contamination was hard to avoid. "One cell from another person, from skin, from breath, or hair, and it will contaminate everything," said Svetlana Milayeva, the Russian geneticist who ran Verlinsky's PCR lab in Chicago. Only the strictest laboratory controls could ensure the purity of the test results.

The most serious obstacle researchers had to overcome concerning the genetic testing of embryos was laboratory conception itself. The failure rate was simply too high to make it practical for any but the most extreme cases. Flaws in the chromosomes and genes of early embryos were considered the major reason that laboratory conception failed so frequently. Australian researchers hoped genetic analysis would help them improve the pregnancy rates by making it possible to sort out the flawed embryos from the healthy ones.

"There is no point in diagnosing embryos if we can't get the woman pregnant when we put it back," said Douglas Saunders in Sydney. "We have to lift our pregnancy rates."

At the Illinois Masonic Medical Center in Chicago, it was called the Virgin Room. No man was allowed to enter. There, secure from contamination by any unwanted cells, Svetlana Milayeva conducted the sensitive PCR assay to determine if an embryo was male or female. A single cell from a male technician could distort the test results.

The DNA thermal cycler she used resembled a cash register. The easiest, and potentially most lucrative, genetic test a lab technician could perform with the human embryo was to determine its sex. If genetic probes for specific inherited diseases proved elusive, the tools needed to detect the presence of sex chromosomes were not. By 1990, researchers had 150 separate genetic probes able to distinguish male from female embryos. It added another twist to the ancient desire to control the sex of offspring.

To conceive a male child, couples once recited chants, and timed their intercourse to phases of the moon or the direction of the strongest wind. Now they used ultrasound and amniocentesis. The technology had changed; the desire for a male child had not. Selective infanticide was the earliest and perhaps most universal form of sex selection. From the Arctic Circle to the tropics, families had taken newborn girls and buried them under rocks, drowned them, or simply let them starve. Monarchs divorced the wives who could not bear them male heirs. During Japan's Tokuwaga period, from 1600 to 1868, some districts routinely reported nine male births for every one female. Historians compared the birth records to the expected ratio of male and female infants and concluded that more than 70 percent of female infants had simply been destroyed.

In modern times, the practice of genetic testing and selective abortion to ensure male offspring was so widespread in some countries it had become a prenatal plague. Since 1982, amniocentesis for sex selection became so widespread in some parts of India—where family pressure for a son was so strong that mothers once poisoned their nipples before nursing a female baby—that the government was forced to outlaw it in public hospitals. Many pregnant women still flocked to private clinics where inexpensive prenatal testing could determine if the fetus they carried was female, and then abort it if it was. Of 50 private obstetricians surveyed in Bombay, 42 said they offered amniocentesis for the purpose of sex selection. Physicians who studied 8,000 abortions conducted in Bombay hospitals during 1986 concluded that all but three involved female fetuses. In Calcutta, more than half the prenatal testing was devoted to sex selection, one survey showed. In South Korea, the practice had become so widespread that the government considered banning all prenatal tests. A majority of women polled in the capital city of Seoul said that if they could not bear their husbands a son, they would not object if the men took concubines.

In Europe and Australia, lawmakers urged that abortion for sex selection be banned. In the United States, where the practice was rare, bills were introduced in half a dozen state legislatures to ban it. The Family Research Council, a lobbying group opposed to abortion, urged the Justice Department to investigate the use of abortion for sex selection. The group called it "a grotesque form of discrimination." It was probably the only thing on which anti-abortion activists and feminists could agree. "Gender is not a disease," said John Fletcher, an authority on biomedical ethics at the University of Virginia. "Sex selection violates the equality between the sexes. It is the start of eugenics."

It was ironic, then, that the most immediate result of embryo sexing was to identify and discard male embryos that might be prone to sex-linked diseases.

On the surface, nothing seemed simpler than the physical differences between men and women, but the actual molecular mechanism of gender was elusive. Until about five weeks after conception, male and female embryos develop identically. Then in male embryos, a genetic switch is thrown that activates a chain of biochemical changes that results in the development of male organs. In the absence of this signal the embryo becomes female. In fact, Adam grew from Eve. The scientists searching for the genes that determined sex hoped to learn how genes orchestrate cell growth, leading to fundamental new understanding of how embryos develop or how cancer occurs. But an embryologist performing genetic testing had only to examine an embryo's chromosomes to determine whether an embryo was male or female.

In the United States, parents already were eager to select a child's sex before conception. Many clinics would prepare special concentrations of a husband's sperm, at $400 a sample, with the promise that it would increase the probability that prospective parents could control the sex of the child they conceived. Each sperm contains only half the genes from the man who produced it, so only half of the sperm cells would contain the Y chromosome capable of spawning a boy. In the average ejaculation, there are slightly more sperm carrying the X chromosome, which results in a girl, but the Y-bearing sperm apparently enjoy an advantage. Even though there are fewer of them, they still managed to fertilize more than half of all eggs. Doctors tried to concentrate the Y-sperm by separating the cells by weight or by how fast they swam. One U.S. doctor patented and franchised his sex-selection technique to "gender selection" clinics that charged $1,200 for each attempt. Conception consumers could purchase gender-selection kits at a drugstore or browse through books on how to choose their baby's sex. There was no shortage of customers. At least twice a week, couples came to Verlinsky's lab in Chicago to choose the sex of their child through special sperm preparations.

In the U.S., doctors claimed a 75 percent success rate for their sperm-selection techniques. In Japan, researchers announced that in controlled tests they were able to produce 34 boys out of 40 births and, in a separate set of tests, 33 girls out of 45 births. Press releases from the Fertility Institute of New Orleans proudly announced the birth of the world's first "sex-selected test-tube baby"—a boy born on January 25, 1986. A year later, the New Orleans infertility clinic announced the first sex-selected test-tube girl. Despite a sustained research effort, there was no completely reliable method for controlling the sex of a child short of analyzing the actual embryo.

The impulse would have been familiar to Greek philosophers 2,400 years ago who first concluded that sperm was responsible for determining the sex of a child. From the right testicle, they believed, came the sperm cells responsible for producing males; from the left came the sperm responsible for producing only females. Their solution to the problem of sperm separation involved a piece of string that could be used to tie off one testicle. Dr. Paul Zarutskie at the University of Washington School of Medicine noted that, in the eighteenth century, French noblemen were advised that surgical removal of their left testicle would guarantee them a male heir.

In the summer of 1990, Alan Handyside sent out his birth announcements. The female embryos he had selected in his Hammersmith Hospital laboratory had resulted in the birth of healthy twin girls. The infants, named Natalie and Danielle, were born five weeks prematurely but seemed to have suffered no ill effects from the biopsy they underwent while only a cluster of cells. The twins were delivered over the weekend. The first Handyside knew of their birth was when he arrived at work on Monday.

"It was an emotional experience to see them. Quite. It's difficult to express," Handyside said. "You see them as embryos. Then you hold them as infants. The transition from cells to an individual is a miraculous event. It gave me pause for thought." Their mother and father had volunteered for the experimental embryo biopsy procedure because she carried the gene for a rare fatal disease similar to muscular dystrophy called adrenoleukodystrophy. Her sister, who also carried the lethal gene, had an eleven-year-old son who was totally disabled by the hereditary disorder.

A few weeks later, the second set of twins was delivered. One was dead. A postmortem revealed no abnormalities. The other twin was healthy. The doctors concluded that the stillbirth was the result of an obstetrical problem. Six other couples, all of whom wanted to avoid conceiving a child with an inherited disease, were also expecting healthy girls.

"This is a staggering success rate that we did not expect," Handyside said. Like Jacques Cohen, he found himself wondering if the hole he had made in each embryo was responsible.

By the fall of 1990, only Handyside and Verlinsky had perfected the art of sexing human embryos. But researchers said the technology would be easy to duplicate in any well-equipped embryo lab. Handyside said he believed that the use of embryo sex-selection techniques was unethical for any purpose except to diagnose an inherited disease. He lobbied actively for legislation to outlaw any other use of the technique, and that summer the British Parliament made it a crime.

Verlinsky's team in Chicago was happy enough to help a couple choose the sex of their child as long as it involved only preselecting sperm. The line was drawn at screening actual embryos. "We would never do an embryo biopsy for simple gender selection, but that doesn't mean that it can't be used for that," said Strom. At least one scientist in Australia who had also perfected the embryo "sexing" in his laboratory refused to publish his work out of fear that the technique would be misused. By the time he announced the first births, Handyside and his colleagues had already persuaded British lawmakers to make it a crime for any doctor to perform embryo biopsy solely to determine a child's gender.

"We managed to convince people it was not ethical to sex an embryo simply so a couple could decide whether to have a girl or a boy. We are doing it only to prevent genetic disease," Handyside said. "Now that we have demonstrated that we can diagnose preimplantation embryos for sex, clinics all over the United States will jump on it. What is to prevent them from doing it simply for sex selection?"

If genes were the family ties that bind, scientists soon sought opportunities to loosen them.

At the National Institutes of Health, researchers began the first government-sanctioned attempts to cure a genetic disease by administering altered genes to human patients. Final government approval was granted at 8:52 A.M. on Friday, September 14, 1990. Barely four hours later, the experiment was under way. A four-year-old girl from Cleveland, suffering from a rare hereditary disorder that left her without a functioning immune system, was infused with one billion of her own white blood cells, to which scientists had added the gene her body lacked. The experiments marked a medical milestone because they were the first successful step toward altering the genetic makeup of an individual. Within two weeks, a private firm called Genetic Therapy Inc. announced that it had obtained an exclusive licensing agreement from NIH to commercialize the techniques used in the first government-authorized attempt at gene therapy. The agreement was announced months before the scientists even knew if their experiment had helped the ailing child.

But the experimental gene therapy at NIH was reserved for only the most hopelessly ill. Without some radical treatment, patients like the young girl could expect to die in childhood. In her case, the researchers tailored white blood cells to carry the healthy new genes. Other researchers experimented with equally exotic ways of improving an individual's genetic makeup. One proposed technique involved expensive and life-threatening bone marrow transplants. Another involved artificial "organoids" of Dacron and Gore-Tex that could function like a gland to release genetically engineered cells into the body. Some researchers were tailoring potent viruses to infect cells with healthy genes. They all had one thing in common: The genetic changes would not affect the sperm or eggs the patient produced. The genetic change could not be passed on to children.

Some inherited diseases so warped the body chemistry of a growing child that, by the time the child was only a few years old, the damage was irreversible. To cure such diseases, scientists would have to intervene even earlier, before the disease had set the pattern of the child's development. The best time, many researchers believed, was when the child was still an embryo. If it worked, the growing child would be free of the disease, and so would all that individual's descendants. Such treatment, called germ-line gene therapy because it involved altering the body's reproductive "germ" cells, would permanently alter the human genetic inheritance.

Scientists routinely altered embryos to create new forms of cattle, sheep, and fish, as Philip Leder at Harvard University had injected genes directly into embryos to create the OncoMouse. They simply forced new genes into fertilized eggs. They injected eggs with microneedles, blasted them with "gene guns," or fused them with electric currents. Perhaps one in 100 would incorporate the new genes and develop normally. The mistakes usually died. Some of the mistakes lived to reproduce. "We have very little control over where these genes land," Dr. Leder said. "Occasionally they will interfere with good genes." In the face of their persistence, the technical hurdles were falling. If scientists could find an efficient way to introduce a new gene into human embryos, they could use the biopsy technique to determine which contained the new gene. If the new gene could not be detected, they could discard the embryo.

Moral and ethical objections overshadowed the technical problems. Prospective parents would have to accept the hazards of a genetic experiment on behalf of a child that had yet to be conceived and, at the same time, give the child the life in which to face the consequences of the experiment. For almost 20 years, religious commissions, medical boards, and congressional panels had debated the idea. "Deciding whether to engineer a profound change in an expected or newborn child is difficult enough. If the change is inheritable, the burden of responsibility could be truly awesome," a presidential biomedical ethics commission concluded in 1982. With the advent of germ-line gene therapy, some physicians argued, medicine would cross a symbolic barrier beyond which doctors were no longer simply treating disease but were involved instead in recreating the human race.

"It will always be considered ethically unacceptable to provide an advantage to a family through germ-line gene therapy, as long as access to health care is not equal. But to correct a disadvantage in a family may be acceptable," said Dr. Jon Gordon, a pioneer in the development of transgenic animals at The Mount Sinai School of Medicine in New York City.

Verlinsky did not plan to wait for gene therapy. Already, he was training physicians for an embryo-screening clinic in

Sardinia to diagnose embryos for a common hereditary blood disorder called thalassemia. He hoped to set up others—to screen for Tay-Sachs disease in Israel, to screen for cystic fibrosis in Europe. "The combination of genetics and IVF is the best way to reduce genetic disorders in the population," Verlinsky said. "In one generation, you could have a healthier population."

In Melbourne, Ian Johnston, the Australian infertility specialist who helped pioneer in vitro fertilization, saw no reason to alter the genetic structure of a human embryo, now that embryo biopsy techniques were available. What couple would assume the expense of risky genetic alterations when they could simply sort through their own embryos and pick out the healthy ones? "I don't know whether genetic engineering to correct abnormal embryos will ever have a place in the human reproduction. It won't in my lifetime," he said. "I don't believe there is a need for genetic engineering in humans now because I think it can be largely overcome by discarding abnormal embryos."

While government officials ignored experiments involving genetic screening of human embryos, they subjected human gene-therapy experiments to the most rigorous public review. Dr. Paul McDonough, the 1990 president of the American Fertility Society, enthused over the potential: To cure an embryo by rearranging its genetic structure was, he said, the "holy grail" of reproductive medicine. And when they finally tried it, they would need human eggs, human embryos. They would turn to those who had learned to shepherd such cells through conception and into the womb.

6

Parents and Other Strangers

Betty Kootz* noticed the blue station wagon in the rearview mirror as soon as she turned out of the driveway at the Feminist Women's Health Center in midtown Atlanta. The man in the orange T-shirt next to the driver was hard to miss. He had been one of the more strident anti-abortion protestors when they first entered the clinic. She turned the car on to Fourteenth Street. The station wagon edged closer. She turned left on to Peachtree Street and sped up to 40 miles per hour. The car stayed squarely in the rearview mirror. It didn't waver as she made a second left turn and circled the block.

"Do you think they're following us?" she asked Sara Weymouth.*

"Surely not," Sara said. "We didn't go in there for an abortion."

She circled the block again and the station wagon stayed close behind. "What do we do? We can't go home. They'll follow us," said Sara.

"I'll do this," Betty replied. She slammed on the brakes so hard that the car almost fishtailed. Unable to stop in time, the station wagon swerved past them.

The man in the orange T-shirt leaned out the window, his

face distorted by rage. "Baby-killers!" he shouted. "Baby-killers!"

In fact, the two women were on their way home to make a baby. Locked in the trunk of their car was a Styrofoam beer cooler containing three vials of frozen human sperm packed in dry ice. It was the middle of September 1989. After years of second thoughts and failed relationships, Sara Weymouth was determined to become a mother. She was thirty-seven years old, and a lesbian. She was deeply in love with her partner, with whom she had been living for more than a year, but, in the eyes of the law and most medical practitioners, she was a single woman. She wanted a child, not a man. She wanted to be a mother, not a married partner. So, she would conceive by herself.

Short, spirited, with Dutch-boy bangs and shins scuffed from weekend soccer games, Sara embodied one extreme. If birth control and laboratory conception had separated sex from reproduction, she represented reproduction separated from sexual identity or preference. "For me, this had nothing to do with sex. It had nothing to do with my sexual process at all," she said. "Reproduction and sex are so coupled in the straight world, but they're not in the gay world. I mean, they don't have anything to do with each other." While Jacques Cohen and his crew of technicians labored in a laboratory to create pregnancies at one end of Atlanta, Sara Weymouth would do it her own way at the other end of town. She needed no high technology, no ultrasound machines, no heightened hormones. All she needed was a syringe and sperm.

She knew the risks. At the moment she made her decision to conceive, she was happily involved with a woman who fully supported her choice. But Sara had to look down the years more bleakly, anticipating the worst. She could not allow herself to assume she could count on the financial or emotional support of her lover, her family, her church, or her community. Sara was open about her homosexuality, but she did not want to be identified publicly as a gay mother. She wanted to raise a child without fear of a custody challenge. Hers would be the only parental name on the birth certificate. She did not want to risk even the remotest possibility of a custody battle with her lover, either. This child would not have two mothers. Her decision to conceive had heightened her sense of vulnerability.

"It is not something you do lightly," Sara said. "There is probably nothing you can do as a gay person that society will censure you more for than to bear a child."

The first time, Sara inseminated herself at the health center. Her partner, Betty, covered her with flowers. Sara rested on a soft pallet in the half-light. Together they chanted prayers.

"It was magical," Sara recalled. She did not become pregnant. At home, she hoped the conception would seem more natural.

That Saturday morning, she traded a letter from her doctor for the vials of semen from the health center. Sara hated the idea of the letter—that she needed anyone's permission to conceive. In Georgia, however, as in many states, it was illegal for anyone but a doctor to perform donor insemination. It was a felony punishable by five years in prison. Her doctor's written consent was Sara's passport to a legal pregnancy.

Almost 80,000 women every year resorted to artificial insemination in an attempt to conceive a child. To most practitioners, a woman's most important qualification for parenthood was her marital status and sexual orientation. About 11,000 doctors offered artificial insemination to their patients, resulting in the birth of 65,000 babies every year, but only one in 10 would inseminate an unmarried woman. There were 400 commercial sperm banks. Reproductive Biology Associates in Atlanta steered clear of single women.

"We have to work within the limits of what the staff will tolerate," said Dr. Carlene Elsner.

When it opened in March 1987, the Feminist Women's Health Center's fertility program was one of fewer than a dozen clinics in the United States that openly offered donor insemination for women regardless of marital status or sexual preference. Women called from as far away as Nova Scotia. By 1990, the clinic had been responsible for six babies. There had been four known miscarriages. There were four women pregnant. About three-quarters of the center's clients were heterosexual; about one-quarter were lesbians. The number of couples seeking its services increased steadily.

For program director Mary Lynn Hemphill and the others at the clinic, donor insemination was, like abortion and contraception, a question of reproductive control. It was the perfect example of a technology women could handle themselves. For lesbian couples, in particular, it offered the only acceptable means of conception.

"As more women can afford to be single mothers and more women have chosen not to marry, donor insemination is just the road they take," she said. "Some women are just wary of the medical system. They often have friends who have been to the depths of infertility work. My younger clients do tend to be gay women."

The National Center for Lesbian Rights estimated that 5,000 to 10,000 homosexual women had borne children into lesbian families and that hundreds more had adopted. As they became more common, tokens of the new family structure surfaced in the mainstream. Newspaper obituaries for the first time recognized two-mother lesbian families. Lesbian custody battles were redefining the laws of parenthood.

In England, where about 1,500 women gave birth every year to children conceived with donated sperm, the British Pregnancy Advisory Service in Birmingham had long accepted single women and lesbians among the 600 women who sought out the clinic's insemination services every month. In 1991, the clinic accepted three virgins as clients. During the ensuing uproar, conservative members of Parliament urged the government to end all fertility services for single women and to ban virgin births. "One virgin birth for eternity is enough," said one British official.

It took Sara Weymouth nine years to decide to have a baby. When she tried to adopt a child, she quickly found that, as a single woman, she was discouraged by most adoption agencies. Then she sought a male friend to act as a sperm donor. "It just didn't seem like an easy thing to go out and locate sperm unless I just wanted to go sleep willy-nilly with whoever would do it with me. It seemed humiliating," said Sara. She did sleep with one former college lover. He was so eager to cooperate that, unasked, he had his sperm count analyzed. She realized that he expected more involvement than she would permit. A homosexual acquaintance offered to marry her and father the child. However, he wanted to share custody. They discussed it earnestly for about eight months before she decided against it. She joined a lesbian "baby-maybe" parenting group to sort out her thoughts. "I didn't want to spend the next several years of my life trying to cook up relationships so that I could have a kid," she said. "I just felt like I was really monkeying with my life."

Donor insemination offered the best solution. "Turkeybaster" babies—conceived with homemade insemination tools—had long been part of homosexual folklore. But now the fear of the AIDS virus made any sample of unscreened semen suspicious and potentially lethal.

Several friends offered to donate sperm. That offered its own entanglements. Biological claims of paternity overrode sexual preferences. Despite a single woman's intention to raise a family without a father, the law often required a child to have one parent of each sex. For the child to receive some government benefits, for example, the mother must divulge the father's name. Even if the child was conceived through artificial insemination, the mother could still be vulnerable to paternity suits. In 1980, a gay man who had donated sperm to a lesbian filed a paternity suit in California court, seeking custody. Three years later, the court ruled that he was the child's legal father and granted him visitation rights. In a similar case, the U.S. Supreme Court turned aside the appeal of an Oregon nurse who did not want to share raising her daughter with the community-college teacher who donated sperm to inseminate her. Under Oregon's artificial insemination law, sperm donors— with the exception of husbands—have no parental rights. A state appeals court had ruled, however, that states may not strip unmarried biological fathers of their parental rights without a hearing.

"What it came down to was that I wanted to get pregnant in the simplest way possible. I debated for years whether to use a known donor," Sara said. "A lot of people think knowing the identity of the biological parent is real important, but to me it feels like a commodity. I think a person's parents are the people who raise them.

"Sometimes I get obsessed about what the kid will look like," she admitted. "Will it look like me? Will it look like someone I've never met?"

Mary Lynn Hemphill warned Sara and Betty in advance to come in the back door. They could expect demonstrators and jeers.

Since the clinic opened as a self-help group in 1977, there had been several attempts to burn it down. Bomb threats were as much a part of the clinic routine as junk mail. More recently, the anti-abortion activists of Operation Rescue had targeted the clinic's abortion service. It took a U.S. Supreme Court decision to clear the path to the clinic's entrance. The doors all had dead bolts. The windows had bulletproof glass. "A lot of the anti-abortion people hate this program a lot," Hemphill said simply.

On Saturday, Sara and Betty were anxious to attract as little attention as possible.

"Bring an ice chest like a picnic cooler. As you go out the door, say something to me about a picnic," Mary Lynn Hemphill told the two women. She arranged the frozen straws of sperm in the cooler and walked them to the car. The demonstrators stared stonily from the sidewalk.

Sara recalled, "We put the cooler in the trunk and I said, 'I'm sorry you can't go on the picnic with us.' "

Mary Lynn Hemphill said in an equally loud, cheerful voice, "Well, good. Have a good time."

Even so, the man in the orange T-shirt was suspicious enough to try to follow them home. When they got inside, they unpacked the cooler and put one vial on the bedside table. "It was white like ice," Sara recalled. "Then it turned clear when it thawed."

She unwrapped a syringe and the clear plastic speculum. She had tried artificial insemination before; she had been pregnant that spring and miscarried after eight weeks. This was the first time she had been able to try insemination at home. She had picked the father from the Caucasian donor list in a catalog. She knew him only by a five-digit serial number. The donor profile mentioned his blue eyes. She liked that.

"You make these decisions completely in the dark. You have to go by your gut. You go with what you are familiar with. You go with what you are hoping for," she said.

She became pregnant. Friends opened a savings account for her expected baby. They helped set up a white-wicker crib and filled it with stuffed animals. There was a bag by the pillow labeled MY FIRST TOYS. Sara saved the syringe.

"I introduce Mary Lynn as the father of my child." She laughed.

Donor insemination—the oldest and simplest assisted reproduction technique—posed some of the starkest questions of reproductive control.

When the technique was used to inseminate a woman acting as a surrogate for another couple, some criticized it as an act of commercial exploitation and reproductive slavery. Others applauded it as an act underscoring a woman's reproductive freedom. Used by a single woman to achieve a pregnancy, donor insemination was an act of biological independence. Others saw it as an act of parental irresponsibility. Sometimes money changed hands; sometimes the procedures were an act of loving charity.

Surrogacy and donor insemination were social and legal arrangements sharing a common technology that offered a biological link to one parent. There was no sophisticated laboratory technique involved in carrying a child for another couple or bearing an infant out of wedlock—only a changing sense of values, class, and contract law. In a formal policy statement on donor insemination and surrogate motherhood, the American College of Obstetricians and Gynecologists warned that "both depersonalize reproduction to some extent. This may affect the particular couple adversely and, with widespread use, may lead to a change in the way society views childbearing."

Here, doctors made themselves custodians of traditional family propriety. No infertility clinic in the United States would knowingly offer its advanced laboratory conception services to a single woman; neither would many commercial sperm banks. Although private physicians accepted four out of every five women who requested donor insemination, their reasons for refusal were rarely medical.

Acting in what they considered the best interests of the child, the conception clinics and sperm banks hewed closely to the most widely accepted social and sexual norms. Doctors routinely turned away unmarried women and lesbian clients as well as women who were "psychologically immature" or on welfare. They also refused women in cases in which they suspected child abuse, drug addiction, alcoholism, or a criminal record. Sperm banks rarely, if ever, rejected men showing similar characteristics who sought to store semen for future use. Those doctors who would accept single women often did so only after psychological counseling. In countries like Brazil, Libya, and Egypt, donor insemination under any circumstances was a crime. A woman who inseminated herself could be arrested and imprisoned. In its code of ethics, the American Fertility Society allowed the insemination of unmarried women.

When researchers from the congressional Office of Technology Assessment surveyed 1,500 physicians and the nation's 30 largest sperm banks, however, they discovered that almost half the doctors failed to follow any of the voluntary guidelines set down by established medical societies. Half said they did not test donors for the AIDS virus. Almost three-quarters did not test for syphilis, gonorrhea, or hepatitis. They also found that many of the doctors who did not screen donor sperm for biological problems—such as viruses, bacteria, parasites, or evidence of genetic defects—did screen donors for other factors, such as intelligence. More than half the doctors thought it was appropriate for them to screen donors for subjective traits such as artistry, creativity, intelligence, and sports ability. The congressional researchers who conducted the 1988 study were baffled by why doctors who spent so little time screening for potentially life-threatening infections would be so anxious to screen donors and recipients for nonbiological characteristics. No one knew how many women or fetuses had been harmed by diseases the doctors overlooked, but the researchers said that their results "paint a disturbing picture."

Clinics in Australia were less concerned about the legal marital status of their clients than about the stability of the household into which a child would be born. By law in Victoria, all prospective couples were required to receive counseling before being admitted to an infertility program. Acknowledging "powerful community disapproval" of providing insemination services to unmarried women, state legal-reform commissions in Victoria, Queensland, and New South Wales recommended that donor insemination be limited to cases "where the mother is married or is living in a *de facto* stable relationship with a man who consents."

In the United Kingdom, where the first test-tube baby was conceived, one survey of physicians showed that more than half believed there should be no screening of applicants. More than one-third believed that artificial insemination should be available for unmarried couples, and a significant minority thought it should be offered to lesbians, as well. Counseling was compulsory under the terms of a new Human Fertilization and Embryology law enacted in 1990. In a country where, by tradition, family is property, parliamentary quarrels over the new law reflected the uneasiness with which many regarded even the simplest techniques for manipulating human reproduction.

Scottish clans and English hereditary peers fought to keep their bloodlines pure by offering amendments that would prevent children produced through donor sperm from inheriting titles, hereditary honors, and coats of arms. So that none would slip through by accident, the peers wanted the birth certificates of those children to be specially marked—a kind of bureaucratic scarlet letter to ensure that no one could mistake the circumstances of the child's conception. In the House of Lords, members sought to prevent unmarried childless couples from receiving any infertility treatment at all. Others tried to make it illegal for a doctor to place an embryo in an unmarried woman. They also sought to bar unmarried couples from licensed treatment centers offering donor insemination. That measure was defeated by a single vote.

One twenty-eight-year-old divorced computer programmer in Sydney was determined to bear her own child, despite local laws that made the artificial insemination of single women illegal. She faxed Mary Lynn Hemphill in Atlanta, declaring her intention to visit the United States, where she could have legal access to donor sperm. She requested information on donor profiles, medical tests, and costs. If she had to return to Australia before becoming pregnant, would the health center allow her to take refrigerated sperm back to Australia? Did the health center know "the position of Australian Customs in this regard?" she asked.

"It is most important to me to obtain a comprehensive character profile [as well as background, IQ level, and appearance] of the sperm donor," she wrote. "Being a single mother," she added, "it may be preferable for me to bring up a daughter. With this in mind, would it be possible for you to increase the probability of me conceiving a child of a certain sex?"

Dr. Sev Rosenwaks riffled through the files in his lap. It was nearing the end of Cornell's daily clinic meeting late in the afternoon of September 19, 1989. He had saved two cases for last. "We have an unusual request," he told the doctors, embryologists, and technicians around the table.

"A woman. Age forty-one. She wants her daughter to contribute an egg so she can have a child with her second husband." The woman had been sterilized after her first marriage. Her second husband had no children. "The daughter is twenty-one and apparently willing." Half of the daughter's hereditary inheritance came from her mother; so the older woman would be genetically related to the donated egg she carried. Rosenwaks looked up from the file. The group murmured its disapproval. The mother would be both mother and grandmother to the child she carried; the daughter would be both mother and sister.

"What would the daughter say when her mother gave birth?" asked one doctor. "This is my baby daughter-sister?"

Another said it had the taint of incest.

"What would it do to the family?" a nurse asked. "Who should the baby call 'Mom'?" This wasn't medicine; this was social engineering, she said.

Rosenwaks enjoyed the stir.

Mina Alikani spoke up. "It's just genetic material," she said.

They turned and stared at her. "The mother passed it to her. The daughter is passing it back." Rosenwaks shook his head. Cornell would pass.

Rosenwaks slid the second folder from the pile. "A woman with Marfan disease wants a donor egg. She suggests her two sisters, thirty-one and thirty-four, as candidates," he said. The hereditary syndrome caused a flaw in the fabric of the body's connective tissues and sometimes weakened the heart. In her case, it was apparently mild enough that she could survive the stress of pregnancy, but she did not want to pass the trait on to her children. The eggs from her sisters would not have the defective gene. Rosenwaks looked around the table. Yes? They would accept her case.

When it became possible in 1983 to transfer human eggs safely from one woman to another, embryologists found they could suspend the biological clock that haunted so many older women. Menopause was no longer a bar to pregnancy. At the University of California in Los Angeles at least four women who had gone through menopause easily became pregnant during 1990 with eggs donated by younger women. In all, seven women over forty volunteered for the experiment. The three donors, women between thirty and thirty-four years old, were paid $1,500 each time they donated eggs. One woman had a miscarriage; one had a stillborn child. But four women previously considered hopelessly infertile delivered normal babies. One had twins. Dr. Marcia Angell, an editor of *The New England Journal of Medicine,* wrote: "The limits on childbearing years are now anyone's guess. Perhaps they will have more to do with the stamina required for labor and 2 A.M. feedings than with reproductive function."

Women could donate eggs the way men donated semen. For women otherwise unable to produce fertile ova, the procedure was the functional equivalent of donor insemination. Any woman could carry another woman's egg or embryo. The technology offered an important emotional advantage over traditional adoption. The man could still contribute genetically to the child, while the wife could experience pregnancy and childbirth. Her links to the child they conceived would be legal and social, not genetic. It would allow the couple to experience pregnancy. Egg transfers could even allow dying women to have their babies born in surrogate wombs. A small but increasing number of women were willing to undergo the pain and surgical procedure necessary to donate their eggs. By 1990, about 300 children had been born worldwide from donated human eggs.

Sperm donors were so common that sperm banks could offer a catalogue of choices, but such was not the case with human eggs. There were no storage vats at hand brimming with extra human eggs. Unlike sperm, eggs were almost impossible to freeze safely. The genetic material was too fragile to survive. Thousands of attempts worldwide with cryopreservation of human eggs had yielded only three healthy babies. When Alan Trounson in Australia performed the first successful egg donation procedure in 1983, clinics used the surplus eggs left over from in vitro fertilization. Once Trounson and Cohen perfected embryo freezing, however, that source of supply almost disappeared. Couples no longer donated their excess eggs. They had them fertilized and froze the embryos instead to give themselves extra opportunities to conceive.

Only by actively recruiting volunteers was Annibal Acosta able to keep the Norfolk donor egg program alive. To solicit volunteers, he met with executives from Planned Parenthood and several large health-maintenance organizations. He was looking for women who had already planned to undergo a tubal ligation. The eggs could be collected as part of the same operation. To his surprise, however, his volunteers turned out to be women simply sympathetic to the plight of infertile women. They were willing to undergo egg-collection surgery as an act of charity. Even more surprisingly, these women recruited others.

"Those donors brought other donors by word of mouth. That was one source that we never thought about," Acosta said.

The clinic screened the volunteers for physical defects and

sexually transmitted diseases, then had them sign a consent form that detailed the risks and conditions of the donation surgery. To produce as many eggs as possible, the donor consented to a regimen of daily injections, daily pelvic exams, sonograms, and blood tests.

"It is understood that I waive any right and relinquish any claim to the donated eggs or any pregnancy that might result from them. I agree the recipient may regard the donated eggs and any offspring resulting therefrom as her own children," read the three-page, single-spaced form. There was a place for the donor's signature. If she was married, her husband also signed it. A doctor and a witness signed, as well. The clinic paid the donor $1,000 to cover the cost of her time. Acosta also insisted each donor be evaluated by a psychologist.

"If there is not some component of altruism, they will be eliminated," said Linda Wilkins, the Norfolk clinic supervisor. "We don't want to feel we are buying their eggs. We also feel it is less likely they will raise questions of parenthood later on," she said. "They never know who the recipient is. They never know if a pregnancy is achieved."

In the fall of 1989, the Norfolk doctors retrieved eggs from eight volunteers. They had rejected four volunteers during the psychological screening; nine others were being interviewed. Each donor, on the average, would provide enough eggs for two women. Up until then, the doctors had transferred 73 embryos made with donated eggs, resulting in 22 pregnancies. Two women miscarried. Seventeen babies had been born. On the average, the women waited two years for a donor. "We try to make a match that will produce a child that will look like a normal product of their normal efforts to reproduce. The best thing is if the woman has a sister. But often they are reluctant to ask. Half the time, they don't want to ask," Linda Wilkins said.

It was the kind of etiquette question only modern medicine could pose. In a café, one woman carefully spooned the froth off her cappuccino and explained the dilemma succinctly. "My friend wanted me to donate eggs." As a mother of two, she said wryly, she was a proven procreative performer. "There's no Emily Post book for this. I didn't know how I'd feel watching the child grow up. It's too complicated. It's too Godlike. I didn't know what to say."

Some said yes. Dr. Georgeanna Jones leaned over the operating table and patted her patient on the shoulder. It was early in the morning on September 26, 1989. The woman had agreed to give her sister what eggs her body could produce. She had signed a donor consent form, designed especially for donation between siblings. In it, the clinic agreed to use her eggs solely for her sister; she waived her rights to the offspring.

"We expect six eggs. She is a little nervous," Dr. Jones said. The experience was painful and disconcerting. The patient's discomfort was not completely caused by the surgery. When she arrived at the hospital, a banner was stretched across the front of the building: GLASNOST FOR SOVIET REPRODUCTIVE MEDI-CINE. Now, as she lay on the operating table, a delegation of visiting Soviet infertility specialists, wearing one-piece white-paper scrub suits and hoods, gathered along the wall. They looked like NASA scientists inspecting a new satellite. A sales executive from Johnson & Johnson served as the Soviet delegation's tour guide. There was no open market yet for the company's fertility drugs in the Soviet Union, but there was no shortage of childless couples or state-run infertility clinics. In the age of *perestroika*, it was never too soon to start building customer goodwill.

Dr. Suheil Muasher, the Norfolk clinic's director of in vitro fertilization, performed the egg retrieval. The procedure was more difficult than usual because the woman had a normal set of reproductive organs, unaffected by endometriosis or cysts. Muasher nodded at the image on the ultrasound screen. "You see the ovary is moving. It is harder to stick. If there were lesions and adhesions, they would hold the ovary in place," he said. A second doctor assisted him. He pushed her stomach with one hand, maneuvering the ovary into position. The woman caught her breath sharply. As Dr. Muasher siphoned the contents of each follicle into a test tube, Dr. Jones wrote the patient's name on it with a blue Magic Marker and handed it through the doorway to an embryologist.

A voice from the laboratory came over the intercom. "We

have one egg." The nurses and Dr. Jones cheered. Hurrah! "We have another one," the intercom announced. The nurses cheered again. The delegation applauded politely, as if they were attending a party rally.

A nurse tapped the woman on the shoulder. "Open your eyes," the nurse said. "Watch the TV set. You can see your eggs."

The woman apologized. "Without my glasses, I can't see a thing," she said.

Dr. Muasher emptied the last follicle and removed the ultrasound probe. The operation was over.

Georgeanna Jones patted her on the foot. "How ya' doing, hon?"

The woman smiled wanly and sipped water from a paper cup as they wheeled her to the recovery area. She had held up her end of the bargain; the family ties were intact.

In the same room barely an hour later, a stranger repeated the sister's act of charity. A volunteer had donated eggs for a woman she would never meet. Doctors synchronized the women's menstrual cycles so that the embryos could be transferred "fresh." The husband and wife signed three separate consent forms. The eggs had been fertilized successfully with the husband's sperm and the resulting embryos were ready for transfer.

The woman waiting to receive the embryos was, by the most common laboratory blood test, male. In all other respects, physically and emotionally, she was female. A rare chromosomal disorder was responsible for her condition. As a side effect, it caused cysts so severe that surgeons had removed both her ovaries. She could not produce her own eggs.

"Hi, there," said embryologist Lucinda Veeck. "Tell me your name out loud." The woman, lying face down on the transfer table, replied. To avoid giving someone the wrong embryos, Veeck made it her practice to repeat the name loudly. Veeck was, to use her own words, "very compulsive" about the embryos in her charge.

She disappeared into the embryo laboratory with the purposeful stride of a natural noncommissioned officer. The door was identified only by a small plaque that read EQUIPMENT

STORAGE. Sperm analysis was conducted behind a door labeled SOILED LAUNDRY. In a moment, she returned holding a loaded catheter veiled in blue-paper wraps. The doctor positioned it. With a gentle push, the embryos were in place.

"You got four embryos," Veeck reported. She held something out in her hand. "Here is a souvenir for you."

The woman looked puzzled for a moment and then she laughed. "Of course. The dish. Thank you."

Altered ideas of family were founded, in part, in the shifting status of women.

Childbearing by single women of all ages had increased rapidly, but there was an especially dramatic rise in the number of older single women having babies. The total number of births to unmarried women in their thirties more than tripled between 1975 and 1986—the most recent year for which statistics were available—and the number of first births to these women increased more than sixfold. In all, there were 2.25 million households run by single women with children.

"It is difficult to account for the rising trend in nonmarried childbearing by relatively older women," federal statisticians noted blandly. "Presumably, many of these women have chosen to become mothers even though they are single."

Sexual equality had demanded unequal sacrifices. Since 1890, the number of women in the U.S. work force had climbed steadily, with an accompanying rise in the average age at which women married, a jump in the divorce rate, and a decline in family size. By 1982, the life expectancy of women leveled off even as the life expectancy of men continued to improve. Women who a century ago might have died in childbirth now died from occupational and stress-related diseases.

Overall, women with children made up half the work force, but they still earned about 66 cents for every dollar paid to men. The number of women working two or more jobs quintupled in two decades, reaching a record high in 1989. Eight of every 10 new employees were women. The higher they advanced, the larger the discrepancy in salaries. In 1990, almost 90 percent of the male executives under forty years of age had children; only 35 percent of their female colleagues could say the same. When fast-track working women put their children first, they found themselves on the "mommy track." When men put their families first, *The Wall Street Journal* approvingly called it the "sanity track."

Outside the workplace, more than half the poor families in the country were headed by single women, their numbers swelled in part by a wave of new no-fault divorce laws. Between 1970 and 1988, the number of single parents tripled to 9.4 million. The number of unmarried couples living together multiplied fivefold. The number of young children living in poverty increased 35 percent. In 1987, for the first time, more women with babies under the age of one were working rather than staying at home. *American Baby Magazine* flourished. *Fathers Magazine* folded.

"I kind of laugh about it because I've always been extremely independent. It just seems ironic that here I am trying to have a kid and basically doing it on my own," said Elizabeth Chandler.* "I must admit I went into it as a very casual, carefree thing. I just assumed it would be a matter of sleeping with somebody."

Procreation did not come so naturally; she had to do it on her own. Every month for two years, she had used donor sperm in an effort to conceive a child. She was single, heterosexual, and she had just turned forty-two. She lived with a man who'd had a vasectomy. He also had a wife, and he showed no signs of divorcing her. Elizabeth sat curled in an overstuffed white chair. It was early December 1989. A fire blazed behind the brass fire screen. She had shoulder-length brown hair and still-water blue eyes. She wore faded blue jeans and a gray cable-knit sweater over a blue cotton turtleneck. She had three university degrees, was a veteran of the Peace Corps and a career in government. She was, for the moment, a dropout.

She always assumed she would have children, but she had always promised herself she would not raise a child alone. She wasn't worried about conceiving a child outside marriage; she was concerned about raising her children outside a stable relationship. She thought she had found the right man. He was clinically sterile. Now she wasn't sure she was capable of conceiving; she wasn't sure she could rely on her partner; she wasn't certain she could simply walk away.

"Much as I would like a child, it's not the end of the world," she said. "Well, some days it is. You get very depressed. I really don't think there is anything wrong with me. I'm just old. My eggs aren't as viable as when I was twenty-five. And at twenty-five, I wasn't emotionally ready to have a child. Sometimes I really resent his vasectomy. There are days I want to run out on the street and grab a man."

She was old enough that the phrase "women's liberation" was still lodged in her vocabulary; old enough to have been buoyed by its rising tide and then caught in its undertow. Her life unfolded against a backdrop of debates about economic equity and reproductive freedom. "I grew up thinking basically that I'd have the house in the suburbs with the white picket fence, except I didn't really want that consciously. I went to a woman's college where you got married when you graduated. I was one of the few women who definitely didn't want that at the time. I really wanted to work, but when I was growing up, my idea of what you did was to be a secretary or something. It wasn't being a lawyer or a professional. Women's lib hit with a vengeance in the sixties and the seventies and I got caught up. I'm not really a women's libber, but just by force of the fact that I wasn't married, I started working and I started moving up the ladder and I just thought I'd always get married. Then you find you don't. And what went along with that was children.

"But I never really thought about having children without a man," she said.

As she approached her fortieth birthday, she considered adopting a child. Her partner persuaded her to conceive; he wanted to see her pregnant.

"I think he really wanted me to have a child. He seems to be very lukewarm to adoption. I mean, he's had children. For him, it's more a question of me having a child—my child—than just a child that we bring up together. I think he wants to see me pregnant. He would like to be the father, but he can't. He knows that. It's been a hard thing for him. He extremely regrets having had a vasectomy. He doesn't want me talking to people about how we're doing it, how I'm doing it. He really, if this child happens, wants everyone to believe it's his child. To the point where he wants to go to the hospital and declare himself the father on the birth certificate," she said. He wanted to claim the child formally, but not their relationship. At his request, she did not tell her family she was using donor sperm.

She started looking for sperm banks in the Yellow Pages. Commercial sperm banks turned her down because she was unmarried.

"I never thought that would even be an issue," she said. "It just really took me aback." One referred her to the Feminist Women's Health Center. She immediately felt comfortable there. She had never liked doctors, and she found the high technology of modern conception clinics offensive. Her best friend was undergoing an exhausting round of reconstructive surgery, hormone treatments, and egg collections at a West Coast infertility clinic. The friend owed her infertility to pelvic infections caused by an IUD. "She absolutely convinced me not to go the high-tech route because I could see what she was going through," Elizabeth said.

If the doctors paid more attention to the subtle rhythms of a woman's body, she believed, they wouldn't need so many ultrasound tests, sonograms, and endometrial biopsies. Even with some of the women doctors she met, there was a macho quality to the technology that put her off.

"Even if the doctor wants to help you, the attitude is, well, do you want to do this aggressively? Are you aggressive about this? I don't have absolute proof, but I think the way I feel is probably just as valuable as some of these medical things. This way is so much less stressful," she said. "I am more in charge of it."

The two of them picked the donor together. Their biggest concern was the fear of contracting AIDS. Two women in Wisconsin and four women in Australia had been exposed to the AIDS virus through donor sperm. Even the most elaborate safeguards seemed ineffective. The wife of a hemophiliac with

AIDS became infected with the deadly virus even after specialists attempted to remove the virus from his semen through separation and filtration. The disease, which so transformed sexual mores in the 1980s, changed the practice of donor insemination, as well. In 1988, the U.S. Centers for Disease Control formally recommended that only frozen semen, following a minimum six-month quarantine, be used for insemination. Some banks, concerned that the AIDS virus could evade detection for even longer periods, quarantined donor sperm for a year. Freezing, however, sharply diminished its ability to fertilize.

Elizabeth Chandler wanted a greater assurance of safety than the guidelines could guarantee. "He was adamant and so was I about not using anything from San Francisco. No matter how carefully they screen people, we didn't really want to have anything to do with that part of the country," she said. For the same reason, he ruled out any donor who had any expressed interest in drama or the arts. "He didn't want any kind of art, which is too bad for me because I would like a child that had some artistic characteristics," she said.

Their caution was justified, if not by the threat of the AIDS virus or the liberal arts, then by the fear of improper record-keeping at the sperm banks themselves. New York State health officials shut down two Manhattan sperm banks after allegations that the facilities impregnated two women with the wrong semen. One white couple alleged that their daughter was half-black. The other woman charged that her child's blood type did not match hers or her husband's. Audits often revealed that clinics neglected to conduct the most rudimentary testing for inherited diseases. Congressional investigators at the Office of Technology Assessment determined that donor semen was sometimes not even tested for fertility. Less than one-third of the commercial sperm banks they surveyed routinely tested for venereal disease and less than half tested for antibodies to the AIDS virus.

Elizabeth Chandler and her partner had only a few lines of type by which to judge each donor. The donor's anonymity was carefully protected. Some doctors routinely mixed semen from different donors to obscure their origin. Others believed that the donors could be protected only at the emotional and medical expense of the offspring, who deserved access to the medical files and family histories of the donors who helped conceive them. The drive for open donor records paralleled the increase in knowledge about inherited diseases.

In Sweden, it had been illegal since 1985 to maintain a donor's anonymity. Doctors were required to keep donor records on file for 70 years so that the children conceived with donated sperm could view them if necessary. Any doctor who failed to comply could be imprisoned. In England, Parliament ordered clinics to keep records of sperm and egg donors for 50 years. In the United States, those who advocated greater disclosure were joined by adoption activists. Most donors were wary of the legal entanglements posed by open donation. Some doctors routinely destroyed all records of a sperm donor to preserve anonymity. But at one northern California sperm bank, donors prepared scrapbooks with their medical and family histories, and even pictures of the houses where they grew up, just in case the offspring of their sperm might one day want to connect with their biological origins.

"Actually, I picked the first donor I used primarily because he was a father of children," said Elizabeth Chandler. "To me, he had proven that he had viable sperm. After that didn't take for a few months, I then switched to somebody who turns out to have been so successful that they've now stopped using him as a donor. Apparently he's fathered too many children." The second sperm donor got her pregnant, but she miscarried almost immediately. Still it gave her confidence in her ability to conceive. She wanted to stay with him. There were other reasons; she liked his grade-point average.

Every morning, she took her temperature to keep track of her cycle. She examined herself to gauge her fertility. When she thought the time was right, she would arrange an appointment with Mary Lynn Hemphill at the health center. She found insemination relaxing; afterward, she would nap. Nothing could be less demanding or disruptive. She could carry it home or take it with her on trips. One vacationing couple arranged for a sperm bank to air-freight frozen semen to each new hotel on their itinerary. One single executive, unwilling to miss an opportunity to conceive, routinely packed her frozen semen in her luggage for business trips. She recalled the first time she carried the plastic ice chest to the airport security gate, wondering whether it could be safely X-rayed.

"Well, what's in it?" asked the security guard.

"Human tissue," she said cryptically.

The guard, thinking her a courier for a transplant surgeon, eyed the warning labels on the ice chest and nodded knowingly. "I see. What organ have you got in there?" he asked.

She thought of her human cargo and what it might become. "All of them," the woman replied.

As the months rolled on, Elizabeth Chandler did not become pregnant. She found herself worrying more about how her child would react to the manner in which she conceived it. "Mainly, I worry that the child would wonder and maybe resent not knowing this other parent," she said. "It's one reason why I feel very strongly about having a father in the picture someday, a person who is a father. My feeling always has been that it may not have to be the biological father. But there has to be a father figure."

She worried about her financial situation. She wondered about her partner. Would he go back to his wife? Would he stay to help raise her child? Could she really trust him, and, if not, could she raise her child alone? The second thoughts multiplied. Every month she drove to the clinic. Another birthday came and went. Now the Christmas holiday was upon her. She thought of going back to work. She was getting too old, she said. When would she have another chance to conceive?

"The problem is that the process takes on a life of its own," she said. "You want to prove to yourself you are physically able to do it. You feel there is something wrong with you when it doesn't take. The more you do it, the more you wonder how anybody gets pregnant."

7

A Piece of Myself
Between Us

I can make life. I just can't keep it," said the thirty-three-year-old market researcher. Dana Hobart* ran her finger around the rim of her glass of iced tea. "I joke I need some Velcro in there, so the embryos will stick in my uterus."

It was a fall day as crisp as an apple. Outside, her husband, John*, thirty-six, trimmed the holly hedges. She sat in the family room, looking at the mantle, lined with baby pictures. It was her gallery of generations; childhood photographs of her husband leaned next to snapshots of her goddaughters and their grandparents' wedding portraits. Dana and John Hobart have never had a child. But for two weeks in the spring of 1989, they kept a color Polaroid photograph in the place of honor on the baby mantle—a microphotograph of two embryos. Theirs. A child's fingerpainting has taken its place, the gift of a friend. The photograph, like the memory of the embryos themselves, was too painful to keep on public display.

Her humor had embarrassed her. She was dark, the youngest daughter of a Southern family, of Italian descent, a lapsed Roman Catholic. A curling mane of coal black hair cascaded down her back. She waved away the wisps that strayed in front of her glasses. In her manner, a shrewd and sophisticated

intelligence mixed with shyness and an old-fashioned reti-
cence—the artifacts of a small-town Southern upbringing.

"I had my little embryo picture up there," she said. "Seeing
those little embryos, and knowing they didn't implant in me,
was devastating to me," she said. "It was the feeling that I
could create life purposely that would almost purposely die.
Its chances were so remote. It seemed cruel, and hard for me
to fathom—creating life only to see it die."

It was a dilemma Dana Hobart never expected when, more
than a decade before, she and her husband first kindled their
dreams of family.

They met at college. She was editor of the school newspaper.
He was president of the student council, a stocky, soft-spoken,
blond Baptist from Atlanta. He showed up at the newspaper
office to invite one of the better-looking reporters to a concert.
Unbeknownst to him, the reporter had other plans that weekend; she was getting married. "She's not available," Dana told
John. She looked him over. "But I am."

Two years later, he proposed in the Greyhound bus station.
She slipped the ring on her finger as they walked to the parking
lot. It was too big. Later, as her father drove them home, she
pretended to sleep in the backseat while John sat in front and
formally asked her father for her hand in marriage.

They wed when she graduated from college. She found work
with a publishing company and started working toward her
master's degree. His business boomed. They moved three
times. They survived sickness, spats, boredom, even success.
More than a decade later their relationship was intact, the
passion still alive.

Dana and John Hobart were proud of their marriage and of
its longevity; they were a shade self-conscious about it, too.
If the years had worn them down, they had worn harder on
those around them. The Hobarts were the only couple from
their college crowd who had never divorced. John's only
brother had been divorced four times. "It makes you want to
work harder to solve your marital problems," John said.

The Hobarts had been married for 13 years, and for the past
six years they had been trying to conceive. She had never been
pregnant. Their doctor diagnosed endometriosis, but, once

that had been treated by laser surgery and hormones, a succession of gynecologists, internists, and infertility specialists couldn't say exactly why the couple remained childless.

"The funny thing about it," Dana said, "is that when we first got engaged, John told me we weren't going to get married until we had five thousand dollars in the bank. I said, 'John, you're crazy.' He had maybe five hundred dollars in savings. Then he said we aren't going to have a kid until we have ten thousand dollars. I said that's crazy, too. We know we want children. We might as well go ahead and do it. About six months after our marriage, we tried to have a baby. Nothing happened.

"We got scared and thought maybe we really are a little over our heads and we should wait. We decided to collect pennies. We said after we have twenty-five dollars in pennies, we would try to have a baby. Isn't that funny? We thought it would take about five years.

"Whenever we were feeling amorous, we'd throw extra pennies in the penny container. And if we had only one or two, we'd say: Baby, you're put off a couple more months there. It was a strange method, but, you know, it worked. About five years later, we really felt we were ready—and we had twenty-five dollars in pennies. I still laugh about it because we are still collecting pennies. We are going to buy a savings bond for the baby when we get enough pennies. That's our goal. Save the pennies and, when we find out I'm pregnant, buy a savings bond. The penny method was very effective for five years. At least I thought that was our birth control," she said.

Dana's parents almost never asked her about grandchildren anymore. Children had become a touchy subject in her parents' household. Dana's older sister never conceived, either, and their mother blamed herself. When pregnant with her first child, she had taken a prescription drug called DES to prevent miscarriage. By 1971, researchers had determined that the drug caused so many birth defects that the U.S. Food and Drug Administration banned its use in pregnant women.

Between 1940 and 1971, doctors prescribed DES to an estimated 4.8 million women in the United States. DES was a postwar wonder drug—a powerful synthetic form of the hormone estrogen developed in England in 1938 and, beginning in 1948, heavily promoted in the United States. In the livestock industry, it was used in feed to fatten cattle and poultry. Among pregnant women, DES was widely taken as pills, suppositories, or injections to prevent miscarriages. Doctors prescribed the synthetic hormone in doses roughly equivalent to 2,000 birth control pills a day. Almost 20 years after the drug was introduced, women learned that its most permanent effects were the consequences for the sons and daughters of the women who had taken it. The drug had somehow crossed the barrier of the placenta to reach the fetus and affect its development after even mild exposures. Researchers linked it to physical abnormalities of the cervix, uterus, and other reproductive tissues. Such women faced a higher risk of ectopic pregnancies, a higher risk of miscarriages, and a greater chance they would be unable to conceive a child at all. Two-thirds of them had malformed uteruses. There also appeared to be cellular changes in the lining of the uterus that made it harder for an embryo to implant. Their bodies were also more likely to produce antibodies to human sperm. In 1990, researchers began to suspect it might be linked to cancers appearing in the generation of grandchildren.

Dana's mother had taken the drug for months during her first pregnancy. As a consequence, Dana's sister was one of the generation of DES daughters. She had already lost one ovary to cysts. She was infertile, and she lived in constant fear of developing cancer. She would require special medical exams and tissue biopsies for the rest of her life. There were an estimated two million DES daughters; about half of them were not even aware of their condition.

Dana may have been the only daughter capable of bearing her parents' grandchildren, but her parents almost never pressured her to have children.

"I only felt the pressure from my family once when my mother and my mother's sister were visiting. When my mother and her sister get together, they reminisce. It's very nostalgic and emotional," she said. "My mother produced this packet of things she had, all my baby things, all our childhood things. She had a little tiny gold bracelet that we had when we were little girls. A little pair of gloves I wore at Easter when I was six. Little baby spoons. What made me feel really bad was she pulled out a clump of my baby hair, light brown. She saved all that stuff. And she presented it to me, saying, 'You can give these to your little girl when you have one.'

"That's when it really got to me. And even then, they didn't really pressure me. It was just that they had all these wonderful memories. They wanted me to have them, too," she said.

Instead of locks of baby hair, silver spoons, or bronzed baby shoes, John and Dana had the photograph of their embryos. It was in a drawer somewhere in the family room. Dana couldn't find it.

Dana Hobart said she doesn't remember when the struggle to conceive became the center of their life. It gathered weight gradually, as their bedside jar of copper pennies filled to overflowing.

Eventually it dictated their diet, their drinking habits, their vacation plans, and their sex life. They bought their first telephone answering machine so that they wouldn't miss a call from their doctor. She bought a digital egg timer to monitor her ovulation tests because the noise of the alarm clock she had been using frightened their dog. She grew accustomed to reaching for a thermometer first thing every morning, to carrying a plastic cup to work in her purse for urine samples, to the needle marks on her hips, to the mood swings, rages, hot flashes, and other side effects of the fertility drugs. She took daily doses of commercial fertility hormones. The Clomid, she recalled, made the world flash around her. When she got up every morning, she would see pinpoints of light dancing in front of her eyes. She said she got used to seeing stars after a few months. Pergonal made her feel like "a lunatic" filled with overpowering rage. "You don't realize how powerful hormones are until you have to take them," she said.

While she was taking Clomid, she reported to the doctor's office every month for an ultrasound scan to make sure the drugs had not caused any cysts to form.

"It isn't as if I feel worthless if I don't have children. It isn't that," Dana said. "It's that there is going to be part of our lives that is missing. There will always be a part that's not complete, like a puzzle with one piece missing. You may be able to tell what the puzzle is and it may look pretty good, but there is that one piece that could make it different, that could make it whole. That's how I feel about it, like there is part of our life that is not quite complete yet."

When, in 1983, the Hobarts first asked their doctor why she had not gotten pregnant, they still weren't convinced there was a problem. Neither was the doctor. "Go home and try again," he told them. "See me in a year."

Two years later, she was back at her gynecologist's with the same misgivings and asking the same questions. She made increasingly frequent appointments with an internist, as well. The temperature charts and tests began. They injected dye into her fallopian tubes to make sure they were open and to check the conformity of her uterus. They snipped tissue samples from inside her uterus. They performed blood tests to monitor her hormone levels. They performed more blood tests to see if she had AIDS or rubella. There were sperm motility tests. John's semen was counted, scanned, centrifuged, and analyzed by computer.

"I don't care what they say, the tests were painful. For the endometrial biopsy, they actually go in with a little curette and grab a part of the lining out of your uterus. It *hurts*. For the other test, they put a metal clamp on your cervix to keep the dye in. Mine kept slipping off and they had to keep sticking it back. It's like—oh, God, please let this be over. Even the sex part was painful because we had been going at it so hot and heavy trying to get me pregnant," she said.

The Hobarts also submitted to a series of postcoital tests. They had to make love and then report to the doctor's office within 30 minutes after intercourse so that technicians could see how well his sperm survived inside her. It added yet another unexpected and unwanted dimension to their sex life.

"The test was scheduled on one of those days when it snowed so badly. We were still trying to get pregnant. We were really going at it. John was so sore. I was sore. We worked like dogs to be ready for the doctor that morning. It was so icy outside that we thought of canceling. But I said: We better do this because I've got it scheduled."

If they could overcome their own modesty and personal squeamishness, they were not going to let something as simple as the weather stand in their way.

"When we got to the clinic, it was closed," she said. "They had closed down the office because of the snow. John looked at me like some kind of dog dragging. But we went back and did the test again," she said.

The Hobarts made the hormone shots, urine tests, and temperature charts a game as best they could. Between themselves, they wore their sense of humor like a kind of Purple Heart. "Things that you normally do in your own bedroom are now being done in little rooms and on stirrups and very sterile surroundings," John Hobart said. He never got used to giving his wife hormone shots. "The first time, I nearly passed out because I was afraid I was going to hurt my wife," he said. "I can't stand to see Dana bleed, so it just drives me wild. It's physically demanding on her, but she never says anything. She never intimates she has a problem."

But each new clinical routine added to the strain. When they fought, it rarely was over credit-card bills or in-laws, but rather over their struggle to conceive a child. And when, discouraged, Dana would tell her husband they should give it up and consider adoption, they fought over that, as well. They instinctively rejected the idea of a surrogate mother. It seemed a prescription for trouble. They would rather try and fail themselves.

"As long as there is a new procedure out there that may allow us to have our own child, I want to try it," said John. "To me that's the ultimate consummation of two people together: to have a little baby that we know are both of us. I want to know what it would be like if we had our own child with all those genes from both of us coursing through that kid's body."

The arguments, he recalled, never seemed fair to either one of them. They had agreed to start on this road together, but they couldn't agree on when to stop.

"She'd say, how many times are we going to do this? Would we consider doing it again if we failed? I said, of course we would. Well, how many times? I said, what am I, an accountant? I don't know how many times, I'm not going to tell you. There are so many factors involved, emotionally, financially. There are so many things that could go wrong and I don't think I should be the one demanding it. I think both of us should be comfortable with it.

"I don't know how many times," John would say. "Until it works."

It was the beginning of the new year and a new patient cycle. In the laboratory at RBA, Michael Tucker was preoccupied. The last cycle of 1989 had been, by general agreement, a disaster.

They could not ignore the numbers. Between Thanksgiving and Christmas, 37 women had come through the operating room. The team extracted and fertilized 252 eggs. From those eggs, they coaxed only 100 embryos. All 100 were transferred into receptive wombs. Only seven women became pregnant. "Hardly anyone got pregnant last cycle, and nobody knows why," said embryologist Sharon Wiker.

In the physicians' changing room, Dr. Massey pulled down his surgical mask and rocked back on his heels. Normally ebullient about the clinic's work, he was somber. "We had a terrible time last cycle. Everything was off. Transfers were difficult. Fertilization was low. My colleagues told me: Don't go into in vitro fertilization if you cannot handle disappointment."

Tucker had come to Atlanta from Hong Kong, where he had been chief embryologist for that city's most successful clinic. Like Jacques Cohen, whom he replaced at RBA, Tucker owed much of his expertise to the IVF clinics in Britain where he apprenticed. He earned his doctorate in mammalian embryology at the University of Birmingham and was chief embryologist for the largest IVF clinic in Britain before moving to Hong Kong. Tucker described himself as a former punk-rocker turned professional baby-maker. For him, the declining birth rate was especially disconcerting. It coincided with his first months as the RBA lab director. No one said it was his fault; not out loud. It could have been caused by a trace chemical in the water, the lubricant in a new syringe, or the dust in the air. One London clinic pinned its barren streak to contaminated oil in the culture dishes. A Houston clinic tracked its poor fertilization rates to gloves worn by the surgeons during egg retrievals. The gloves were powdered to make them easier to pull on, but the powder poisoned the eggs and sperm.

The lab work was a discipline of details. "There are times when you go through a patch where you get paranoid," said embryologist Graham Wright. "We changed everything—all the disposable plastic goods, all the chemicals." Tucker ordered new supplies from the manufacturers, making sure the orders came from different factory batches. They changed the gas tanks. They bought new mineral oil. They arranged to buy syringes from a different supplier. They checked the water—already screened through six separate filters for minute traces of poisonous chemicals. They even looked for changes in the electrical resistance of the water. Still not satisfied, they double-checked the temperatures of the hot plates under the microscopes. The temperatures of the incubators. The temperatures of the hot blocks that held the test tubes. Then they crossed their fingers and checked everything again.

The declining birth rate would drive the patients to other infertility clinics. No matter how diligent the embryologists were in their work, there sometimes wasn't anything for anyone to find, no discernible reason, no rhyme. When IVF Australia in Port Chester, New York, published its weekly fertilization rates, the chart's abrupt zigs and zags looked like wild stock market swings of speculative fever. Nonetheless, RBA's flagging birth rate was Tucker's problem. It weighed heavily on all of them.

For a moment, the doctors found themselves in the same position as their patients. They couldn't get pregnant and they didn't know why.

John and Dana Hobart joked that the house was too big for themselves alone, about wallpapering children's rooms they might not ever need. They shook their heads at the other couples they sometimes saw in the clinic waiting room, the husbands and wives who sat side by side like strangers in an airport—not touching, not talking, avoiding each other's eyes. They read up on the medical procedures. John talked it over with his barber. They tried to involve their families, but it became a secret they could share most easily between themselves.

John recalled, "I put on a videotape of her laser surgery for her father. After two minutes, he just got up and walked out. He couldn't stand it. I was looking at it as basically a medical procedure, but he was looking at his daughter."

If there was to be consolation, they would have to find it in each other. Some days the jokes were too bitter to be borne. The anguish became anger and the arguments exhausted them both. Neither felt the other really understood the pain. They reached for support and found themselves off balance. A single word hung in the sullen silence between them: *children.* It was a word that had been rubbed raw. It revealed something different in each of them.

"Dana," he would tell her, "the difference between us is that you want a child. I want *our* child. I'll adopt if we have to, but I want our child. As long as there is a new procedure out there that may allow us to have our own child, I want to try it."

When she said adoption, he only heard surrender. In her own mind, adoption meant release. "Whenever we bring it up, there is immediate hostility," she said. "Immediate tension between us whenever we talk about it. We don't fight, but there's this wall that goes up immediately. Part of me gets upset because I think how much does he really want me to go through before he realizes that I can't go through any more? There's not that much left of me to endure."

For John, it was bewildering. They had pledged their troth in sickness and in health; this was neither. Their life was full and hollow. "Dana never had even a cold, and all of a sudden we're faced with this issue of infertility. It's not a big disease. It's not like cancer, but it can be as emotionally stressful. Probably more so, because we can't find any causes. I think it was a year and a half she was saying she had a problem, and I was saying no, it's just a matter of having sex more often."

At Thanksgiving, they tried artificial insemination again. Before they could tell if she was pregnant, they went on a vacation cruise. They sunned themselves on the Caribbean halfway between San Juan and Barbados.

"It was expensive," John said, "but it was cheaper than IVF." And for them, no more effective.

Dana was increasingly unsure whether she had the courage to try again. Finally, one Saturday morning, something inside her rebelled. She awoke and reached automatically for the thermometer. She stopped. *This is another month wasted on a futile attempt. I am not getting any younger. This is really going nowhere,* she thought.

"What scares me about all this is that I'm such a patient, plodding person that I may not realize what this is doing to me in the long run. I may wake up one day and be a total vegetable."

That day, Dana and John buried themselves in chores. Neither spoke. The words churned within her, then overflowed.

"Look, I can't go through this much longer," she pleaded. "This is killing me. You have to help me with this. I have to know if you don't want to adopt. I have to know now. If you do, fine. If you don't, fine. I have to know it because it is killing me. It's killing me knowing that I will never have a child. If I know the answer now, I can cope. But I can't cope like this."

John listened. He didn't have an answer. He didn't have an answer for three days. Then one evening he sat down with her. "I've been thinking hard about it, and I want you to know I will adopt when we have exhausted all our alternatives," John said. "I would love that child just as much as I would my own. But there is a part of me, Dana, that really wants my own child.

"I know you have had it worse than I have," he told her. "It kills me when they put you up on that table. It kills me when they monkey around inside you. I can't stand seeing you in pain. I can't stand seeing you worried about everything. I can't stand giving you shots.

"We'll try one more time, and if you really don't want to try anymore, we'll adopt. I don't want to keep putting you through this," he said.

For Dana, the words opened doors. "Up until that point, I never knew how much it meant to him. He really wanted his own child, his flesh and blood, his own mistakes, his own successes. I guess I should have known that men felt that way, but I didn't. I didn't think it would be that important. Maybe because I am a woman I look at it a little differently.

"It calmed me in a way," she said. "I think our marriage has gotten better because of this. I also see that if we continue on this path without resolving it together, there will come— maybe not a breaking point, but a changing point in our lives where we're not going to be the same people we were. We're not going to have the same relationship. I don't want that to happen."

After $12,000 in medical bills, half a dozen ultrasound tests, laser surgery, sperm tests, three attempts at artificial insemination, and dozens of hormone shots, Dana and John Hobart had agreed to try again.

They were so impressed with the preliminary pregnancy results from Jacques Cohen's hatching experiment that they volunteered for the January experiment—anything, they decided, to improve their chances. They signed the consent form. She got a prescription for the antibiotics and steroids required prior to microsurgery.

Tucker felt the eyes on his back. Jacques Cohen had returned to RBA as a scientific consultant. The visit to the laboratory was cordial; the two were old friends. Its unspoken purpose was quality control.

Cohen stood uncomfortably in the center of the crowded room, his hands clasped in front of him, a stranger in the laboratory he controlled only a few months before. Every time they cleaned it now, they removed another piece of him. The tabloid headlines and the bumper stickers were disappearing. There were hugs and hellos. Everyone was smiling. Everyone was tense. In the silence, the roar of the air conditioning was deafening. "I'd forgotten about the noise," Cohen said. His eyes weighed everything.

Like his Atlanta colleagues, Cohen had found himself with little to celebrate at Christmas. His hatching experiment at Cornell had gone awry. Pregnancy rates had dropped dramatically. Burglars stole the telephones in his research lab. "Cornell has had a bad streak," embryologist Mina Alikani would say guardedly to colleagues. "Lots of transfers and few pregnancies." Cohen performed microsurgery on embryos for 13 women in a row, but none became pregnant.

It was worrisome. Cohen and the Cornell IVF unit was part of a self-styled star system at New York Hospital. The hospital administrators were counting on his performance to help restore the institution's eroding prestige, tarnished by a grand jury investigation of one patient's death that found "woefully inadequate care." The hospital had budgeted more than $5 million in annual operating costs for the IVF program. Administrators expected the IVF program to earn that much and more in community goodwill. They wanted happy new parents spreading the word throughout New York, not declining success rates.

For Cohen and Massey, the falling birth rate at the two clinics was especially disturbing. Despite the success of the first three clinical trials, they were worried that Cohen's new "hatching" microsurgery might be to blame.

Massey had crowed that the microsurgery might push the clinic's pregnancy rate to more than 30 percent—the best in the world. Instead, the pregnancy rate plummeted. Only a month before, he was prepared to offer the new technique to every new patient. He called it a "revolution," and urged his colleagues to adopt it as clinical routine. When he explained it to patients, he wore the contented smile of a man happily surfing the wave of the future. Now Massey, Cohen, and Tucker stared gloomily at the patient statistics for December. Massey went back to the patients and told them that his predictions were premature.

They had other reasons for second thoughts. The first of the women in the hatching experiment had just delivered twins more than nine weeks premature. The mother had suffered other complications that threatened the pregnancy. Doctors induced labor early. Her twins were born, weighing one pound and two pounds, and died within hours. There was no reason to blame the microsurgery; it was just a bad omen. But the hatching pregnancies had yet to produce a healthy baby. It would be several months before they would know the real outcome of their embryo experiment.

Cohen shook his head ruefully. "I know hatching worked in Atlanta. Things are different at Cornell. Here it worked. There I don't know if it works. The culture medium is different. The embryo transfers are different, more forceful, more traumatic. We get a little blood in the catheter," he said. He had already moved to revamp all the laboratory procedures. Cohen suspected that part of the problem was the layout of the hospital itself. A busy hallway—crowded with lockers, medical-waste bags, and nurses from other wards—separated the microsurgery room from the embryo laboratory. After every hatching procedure, Cohen and Malter had to carry the altered embryo through the open hallway. "I don't feel like running across the hall with embryos and running into people," Cohen said. "I've bumped people twice. No harm was done, but something will happen eventually."

Major laboratory renovations were now under way at Cornell. The building was filled with men wielding jackhammers. "We are worried about how construction will affect things. The dust. This is very delicate," said Sev Rosenwaks. He pasted a star on the wall calendar to mark another pregnancy.

"Oh, do jackhammers affect embryos?" asked Dr. Alan Berkeley, Cornell's director of gynecology.

In the embryo lab, the phone rang for the fifth time in twenty minutes. "No, we don't do air conditioning. We do embryos," snapped Alexis Adler, and slammed down the receiver.

At the microscope, Mina Alikani rubbed her eyes. "I think I'm going blind," she said.

Until the carpenters and plasterers finished, Cohen refused to do any more embryo microsurgery. He urged the Atlanta doctors to hold up their own trial until they could reestablish their pregnancy rate.

After the initial euphoria, caution was asserting itself. They had already decided that more clinical trials were necessary before adopting embryo surgery as a routine. "We want to make it more scientific," Tucker said. Even before they secured permission for the experiment from the Emory University human medical investigations committee, the Atlanta doctors already had their nurses recruiting 100 patients for it.

But by the second week of January—when Dana Hobart was scheduled for in vitro fertilization there—RBA's pregnancy rate was so bad that they questioned the wisdom of even a limited experiment. Who could tell whether there was a problem with embryo microsurgery when the doctors weren't even sure the laboratories could get anyone pregnant?

"Wait a month. Wait three weeks," Cohen urged Tucker. "Wait until you know you are getting good pregnancies and then start the hatching experiment again." Tucker stared at the floor. "Is that a problem?" Cohen asked.

"Well, the nurses will have to row back with the patients," Tucker said quietly. "They've all been told they can participate in the experiment."

Cohen was impatient. "So what?"

Tucker kept his eyes studiously on the floor. "Well, the problem is that the patients have really taken hold of this. They really think it is the greatest thing since sliced bread."

Cohen insisted. "Just don't tell anyone. It's a controlled trial. Say they have a fifty percent chance of having their embryos hatched and then don't do it. Just wait a few weeks," he said.

Massey joined the argument. "The first thing is to do no harm," he drawled. "It won't kill us to stop hatching for a couple of weeks to make sure we are back on track again. We have to tell the patients. We've already told them we are doing hatching on every other patient."

They agreed in silence. "Well, we have progressed," Cohen said. "We have progressed in what we understand. I really thought it was such a simple thing—just a hole in the embryo. Maybe I am wrong."

"I really thought hatching would take off," said Massey.

"So did I," said Cohen. "I have had sleepless nights about that."

The aftertaste of crow was bitter. In the lab office, a stuffed effigy of "The Boss" had been pinned to the wall like a voodoo doll, stabbed through the heart with a nine-inch egg-collection needle. A new tabloid headline found its way onto the office door: MOM'S TEST-TUBE BABY IS THE WRONG COLOR! WE'RE STILL IN SHOCK . . . THE CLINIC MADE A *HORRIBLE* MISTAKE!

Dana Hobart surprised herself. For the second time in a year, she stretched out on an operating-room table wrapped in blue surgical drapes and stared at the ceiling while Dr. Hilton Kort probed her ovaries for the mature eggs they harbored. The steady rise and fall of her pulse and respiration were traced in amber and green waves on the instruments next to the anesthesiologist.

She hoped the new year would be a lucky one. Out of the corner of her eye, she could see the video monitor and the image of her uterus projected by the ultrasound probe. The black-and-silver image shivered like sunlight filtering through ocean depths. She was the first patient that morning. Four more women waited.

"First follicle on the right," called the nurse, opening the hatch between the operating room and the embryo laboratory. Kort probed for the first egg. On the ultrasound screen the black sphere of the follicle collapsed like a punctured balloon. The nurse handed a tube of bloody serum through the hatch.

"I'll just kick off then," said Tucker. He splashed the contents of the tube into a shallow petri dish, swirled it in the green light under the microscope. "A few cells. No egg." Another tube passed through the hatch. Then two more. "Still no egg," Tucker said. He tossed the dishes into the medical-waste bag. Jacques Cohen bobbed over his shoulder, watching. Two more tubes. Nothing. "Just a lot of blood coming through," Tucker said under his breath. A thicket of empty test tubes sprouted between the fingers of his right hand. "Nothing."

With the pipette, Tucker singled out an infinitesimal swirl of cells. He peered intently through the microscope.

"Okay, one egg," he sang out. Quickly he moved the egg into a second dish, rinsed it, then lifted it into a small drop of mineral oil floating in a third dish at his left hand. He placed the last dish under a glass hood and turned back to the microscope.

Kort quickly drained each follicle with the aspiration needle. New tubes passed through the hatch.

"One egg in that last follicle," Tucker called.

Cohen watched from the corner.

Abruptly, the hatch slammed shut. Barely 30 minutes after it began, the harvest was over. In the operating room, the overhead lights came on. The nurses lifted Dana Hobart onto a wheeled gurney and rolled her out of the room. Eleven tubes of fluid were drained from follicles in the right ovary; 17 tubes from the left. Tucker found six eggs in all. "One came through in the wash after they closed the hatch," he said.

John Hobart thumbed through a magazine in the waiting room. Earlier, just after 7 A.M., he had entered the clinic's "masturbatorium." A few minutes later, he delivered his semen sample to the clinic's front desk.

In a cramped office next door, Sharon Wiker slid the sperm sample into a small computer. Sensors automatically measured the speed of each wriggling cell by analyzing the shadows cast by the sperm heads. On the tiny monitor, each head blazed as if it were composed of pure light. The computer reported 51 million cells per milliliter. Three-quarters were moving. It was an electronic parlor trick. The computer actually counted only 93 cells, averaged the results, and then made a programmer's educated guess.

In the waiting room, John Hobart felt discouraged and tired. His grandmother had died; he had flown straight from the funeral to the clinic. His sinuses were stuffed. "I'm not a gambler," he said. "I don't really believe this is going to work."

Michael Tucker finished the last of his bacon, lettuce, and tomato sandwich, wiped a fleck of mayonnaise from his cheek, and then, after changing into faded-green surgical scrubs, did in a minute what Dana and John Hobart had been unable to do by themselves in 13 years of marriage—fertilize an egg.

It was an act that did not require their presence. As John Hobart frowned over contracts in his office and Dana Hobart napped at home 15 miles away, Tucker, following a familiar recipe, assembled the ingredients for life in the womb kitchen.

With a clinician's sleight-of-hand, he uncapped a test tube of John's sperm, waved the open mouth over a spirit lamp, slid a shallow dish out of the incubator, and checked the name etched on its underside. Certain then of the identity, he located the eggs under the microscope, each isolated in its own clear drop. With a sterile pipette, he added a concentrated droplet of John Hobart's sperm. One, two, three, six eggs in all.

Tucker dropped the pipette into an orange medical-waste bag and returned the dish to the incubator, where it would bake overnight at body temperature. He noted the time on a lab sheet and clicked his tongue in concentration. There were other embryos yet to freeze, eggs to collect, an embryo transfer later that afternoon.

Dana Hobart was testy on Thursday. Everyone in her office had questions; she seemed to be the only person who had answers. She could barely concentrate for wondering about her eggs.

Already she had called the clinic once that morning to double-check the dosage of the steroids and antibiotics she had been prescribed for the hatching experiment. She continued to take them even though the experiment had been postponed for several weeks; no one told her to stop.

She hoped at least for a hint about her eggs, but the nurse said there would be no word from the laboratory until after four o'clock. It was still only 2:30. "It's the biggest hurdle," she said. "If they don't fertilize, then nothing can happen." The phone rang. She lifted it from the cradle, ready for an impatient executive's bark.

A woman's voice asked, "Mrs. Hobart?" It was the clinic. "Well, we've got fertilization and we want to see you at the clinic tomorrow at two-thirty P.M. for the transfer. How are you feeling?"

"Sore," Dana replied. Only then did she realize she had been holding her breath. "Well, I am thrilled." *I think I'm running a fever,* she thought to herself. No one would tell her how many eggs had fertilized. She was still unsure how many eggs had been retrieved from her ovaries the day before. The nurses kept saying five, but the lab records showed six.

"If we have to wait any longer, the embryos will have grown up. They'll be able to walk over here and climb in," said John Hobart, looking at the wall clock. It was four o'clock on Friday and they had been at the clinic since 2:30. For more than an hour, his wife had been lying on the examination table where she would receive their embryos, a white wool blanket draped around her legs. He sat nearby on a stool. Dr. Kort had scheduled the transfer for three o'clock, but had been delayed by another patient.

"Are you comfortable?" asked the nurse. "You don't look comfortable."

"I'm fine," said Dana. "I have to hang around here. John has my underwear." The silence stretched on. "I'm sleepy," she said. She pulled the blanket up around her shoulders. A violin concerto played on the radio in the laboratory next door, underscored by the mechanical wheeze of the embryo-freezing machine.

In the doorway, Sharon Wiker appeared, dressed in paper cap, mask, and plum-colored scrubs. She dropped the mask. "You have five fertilized eggs, five embryos," she announced. "They are beautiful embryos. We always freeze the nicest-looking ones. We froze two this morning—two four-cells." Only one egg had not fertilized.

Dana sat up eagerly. "I'm officially excited now." She beamed at John. "I've been holding it back. I feel great about five out of six eggs fertilizing. That is such a miracle."

John looked at her bleakly and deliberately denied the hope in her eyes. "Wasn't it Caesar who had someone ride behind him in his chariot to remind him all his conquests could vanish?" He shook his head sheepishly, embarrassed at his eagerness to anticipate failure. He only wanted her to stay calm. Throughout the weeks of hormone injections, John had been relentlessly optimistic, while Dana had been constantly depressed. Now that they had arrived at the moment of the embryo transfer, they switched roles. John shied away from the idea of success; Dana, for the first time, was at last willing to embrace it.

The TV monitor flickered into life. Three embryos appeared on the screen, floating in a curve like a living archipelago—one four-cell embryo, one five-cell, and one eight-cell. John stood in front of the screen and stretched out his hand, like a new father about to tap at a nursery window to wake a sleeping infant. "The four- and the eight-cell are very beautiful," said Sharon Wiker. "The five-cell is, well . . ."

Dana and John Hobart were transfixed by the television screen. In that moment, what did they see? Three gray translucent clusters of cells. The future. Continuity. A family portrait. Their own image unveiled. Something that bloomed in the empty place inside themselves. Could they even know? "What in this context is beautiful?" John Hobart asked carefully.

"You look for fragments," said Sharon Wiker. "The five-cell has quite a few fragments in it. It is not as nice as the others."

"They can look like the milkman for all I care," said Dana, hugging her knees.

"If they look like the milkman," said John, "I'll sue." Then he laughed.

Sharon Wiker stepped back across the threshold into the embryo laboratory and pulled her gauze mask back into place. "They are always so paranoid about someone misplacing the sperm," she said. "They always say something sarcastic." She donned a pair of sterile surgeon's gloves and prepared the embryo catheter for transfer.

"Are we ready?" Hilton Kort had finally arrived.

Two catheters lay bent and bloody on the instrument tray. Kort held up a third, its plastic tip bright with blood. "I don't want to waste these embryos," he said. "These are beautiful embryos. I don't want to waste them. I'm sorry. I really tried."

Dana put her hands over her eyes. The tears would be for later. Her feet were still cupped in the stirrups. John pressed his forehead against the examination table in an attitude of prayer. The room was dark. The only light came from Kort's high-intensity headlamp.

For 35 minutes, Kort had attempted to thread the looping plastic catheter through the eye of her cervix, to place the three embryos near the entrance of her fallopian tubes, where the fused gametes could resume their interrupted journey. For 35 minutes, Kort tried and failed to navigate her twisting anatomy. The catheter tip snagged repeatedly on the folded tissue of her uterus. Twice Kort returned the apparatus back to Sharon Wiker and ordered the embryos transferred to new, stiffer catheters. "I'm sorry. I've bent a few catheters in my time. We want to be sure the embryos go where they are meant to go. I'm doing my best not to hurt you," he said.

"You're not hurting me at all," Dana Hobart said. She bit her lip, but not in pain.

"Embryos are pretty resilient, by the way," Kort said. "We used to rush to get them back in. We would rather spend the extra time getting them in properly."

Sharon Wiker slipped into the pool of light with the last catheter—the stiffest available. Gamely, Kort adjusted its tip and tried again to feed it into Dana Hobart's uterus. She lay motionless, feeling only the pressure of the catheter inside her, in a condition for which there is not yet a name—in a state of suspended pregnancy, with three embryos marooned on the far shore of her birth canal, denied the safe harbor of return.

"There is blood in your cervix now," Kort said. His shoulders slumped. "Even this is not going in. It's not going to budge." The cervix was tightly closed. The cervical canal hooked sharply to the left. Kort looked up at her quizzically. "Did your mother ever take DES?" he asked abruptly.

"Yes," Dana said. Her voice cracked. "But only for a few weeks. She took it longer for my sister." Kort had voiced her fear—that her mother's medication had reached across the years and marked her, just as it had touched her childless, older sister. "My mother told me she had only taken it for two or three weeks. I've told all my doctors that my mother took DES. None of them ever thought it mattered."

Kort held up the catheter where she could see it clearly in the light. "You expose the embryos to that blood and I can guarantee you won't get pregnant. I think these embryos should be frozen and we should try to dilate your cervix next month. If we can't do that, we should return the embryos surgically," Kort said.

Kort sounded confident, but he was already worried about other complications. Not all embryos survived the freezing process. One of the three embryos was already too far advanced to be frozen safely by the conventional technique. The lab would have to keep it in culture for another three days until it reached the blastocyst stage, when they could freeze it safely in a glycerol-based antifreeze. Left outside the womb that long, three of every four embryos usually died. Even if the embryos survived, they could, because of her DES exposure, implant themselves improperly. If that happened, the result would be a painful, and potentially lethal, ectopic pregnancy.

Kort took their silence for assent and snapped off his gloves. "We are going to have to baby-sit your embryos for a while," he said.

8

Selling the Stork

Overnight, the sales teams transformed two floors of the San Francisco Hilton into a carnival of commercial conception.

In the aisles winding through the temporary sales booths, detail men passed out sperm-shaped wall magnets, condoms imprinted with corporate logos, ovulation kits, and pocket-sized birth-date calculators. Others urged doctors to burn holes in grapefruit with the newest surgical lasers. Companies hawked high-performance semen analyzers, precision cell freezers, and echo-tip ultrasound needles.

Gathered under company banners at the forty-fifth annual meeting of the American Fertility Society, sales reps pitched the high technology of conception like sideshow barkers. PREGNANCY IS POSSIBLE! declared the brochure from Sandoz Pharmaceuticals Corp. LIVING PROOF! the headline promised. TURNS HOPE INTO REALITY! In finer print, the pamphlet noted: NO INCREASED RISK OF MULTIPLE BIRTHS OR FETAL ABNORMAL-ITIES. In full-page program ads, Ares-Serono Inc., which sold fertility drugs in 75 countries, solemnly proclaimed: WE ARE CREATING THE FUTURE.

In its sales handout, Tambrands Inc. assured physicians that its home ovulation kit "is changing the way women have babies." The company also promised "heavy advertising and promotional support" with "millions of dollars in advertising via television and print resulting in 58,000,000 consumer exposures." Couples would seek out the product on their own; the doctors would only have to scribble the prescriptions. And if that seemed like too much work, one firm gave away prescription pads with the name of its product already preprinted on each form. As part of its promotional literature, a second company passed out forms listing the proper insurance code for each of its products, to ensure that no physician overlooked an opportunity for payment.

For the 2,600 doctors, nurses, and embryologists who flocked to the annual fertility meeting, the trade booths were treated as an afterthought. The medical professionals didn't like to be reminded of just how much the womb had become a marketplace. But the money to be made was enough to make the most solemn small-town practitioner giddy. Sales of "First Response" ovulation prediction kits, for example, went from zero in August 1985 to about $15 million annually 24 months later. The salesmen and the doctors each sought to expand their business by encouraging couples to adopt the new technology. Together they were marketing hope to prospective parents. The only question was: Whose brand?

There was nothing new about medical marketing. In magazines and television, doctors routinely pitched liposuction, breast-enhancement surgery, eating-disorder clinics, and employee drug-counseling services. What was unusual about the commerce in conception was the degree to which—in the absence of any federal support or control—commercial interests shaped the treatment of infertility and influenced the direction of research into human reproduction.

Nowhere has the new technology of reproduction been so successfully commercialized as in the United States. Many of the newest medical advances in laboratory conception were imports: The first test-tube baby was born in England; embryo freezing was first successfully performed in Australia and Holland. American men and women quickly became the world's most avid consumers of infertility services. But as long as the federal government was unable, or unwilling, to pursue such research, infertile couples in the United States paid the high cost of disappointment. Or—as was more often the case—they paid for the experiments themselves.

It was, in the strictest sense, free-market science driven by patient demand and willingness to pay. Not only did patients pay more, but, as consumers, they were forced to run greater risks. Throughout the decade, embryo labs were exempt from the state and federal medical-licensing requirements. The public agencies that failed to protect consumers also did nothing to safeguard the infertile men and women who volunteered for embryo research. None of the federal regulations or safeguards addressed experimental techniques designed to enhance a particular couple's procreative choices. And the government did equally little to ensure the health of the children the laboratories had conceived.

Only a few companies sold the hormones or provided the equipment. Often, they were the sole outside source of research funding. They sponsored the professional symposia and paid for the training seminars, organized patient education meetings and funded patient support groups. In some cases, they owned the clinics that set the international standards for proper practice. They even wrote the textbooks. To a remarkable extent, the companies controlled the environment in which the doctors practiced their specialty and patients pursued treatment. The research they encouraged usually demanded more, not less, of their expensive technology. When sales leveled off, company executives were known simply to rewrite a product data sheet, which specified the accepted clinical applications of the drug, to expand use of an existing fertility remedy to a wider group of patients. If the doctors wouldn't pay attention, the companies would seek out the patients on their own.

The marketplace, harnessed to the vested interests of drug companies and the medical community, enforced an orthodoxy that often served as a passive barrier to innovation, even in a field that moved as rapidly as laboratory conception. In the absence of outside research funding, commercial interests fostered experiments that would lead to higher sales or that would require greater exercise of medical control over conception. No one actively sought to exclude other ideas; there was simply little professional or economic incentive to adopt them. A doctor's professional fear of failure and the commercial drive for profit could be obstacle enough.

Inventive medical marketeers walked a legal tightrope. On the one hand, once the federal government approved a new drug for market, physicians were free to prescribe it for any use they chose, regardless of the government's original grounds for approval. A physician could—and often did—prescribe a cancer drug to treat infertility or to cure endometriosis. What a doctor was allowed to do, however, a drug company was not. To protect patients and consumers, the U.S. Food and Drug Administration placed strict limits on what a pharmaceutical firm could encourage others to say about unapproved uses of its products or newly emerging scientific information about them. To sidestep such regulations, companies often sought shelter behind third parties, disguising promotion campaigns for unapproved treatments by funding education seminars and brochures prepared by an ostensibly independent group. In theory, that relieved the company of any legal liability. "We're beginning to see a lot of artificial programs and publications that are a joke," one senior FDA official said.

In March 1990, the FDA formally censured the manufacturer of Lupron for its attempts to take shelter behind an independent organization called Reproductive Education and Choices for Health (REACH). The health group was promoting the anticancer drug, sold usually at about $105 a kit, as a treatment for endometriosis, a leading cause of infertility. In a five-page "Notice of Adverse Findings," FDA's acting director of Drug Advertising and Labeling division, Kenneth R. Feather, declared that the agency was "strongly opposed" to any firm's creating, distributing, or funding any activity that would encourage consumers to try unapproved uses of a company's products. "We are even more concerned when the activity overtly promotes administration of the sponsor's product for the unapproved use, as in this case," he wrote. "We were also concerned by the direct dissemination of the brochures by patient groups as well as by physicians who had elected to administer the drug for these unapproved uses . . . If the brochure is disseminated directly by a patient group outside of the physician-patient relationship, it only creates demand for an unproven therapy." Not until October 1990 did the company gain formal FDA approval to market Lupron as a treatment for the 5 million U.S. women who suffered from endometriosis.

In the conception business, where dreams were the yeast that leavened rising profit curves, the drug companies adroitly promoted what one sales executive called "fetalmania."

No single corporation dominated the field more than a pharmaceutical firm owned by the Bertarelli family in Italy.

The Ares-Serono Group, a multinational corporation that produced four of the most common prescription drugs used to treat infertility, was the foundation of the family's $1 billion fortune. Until the early 1970s, the Vatican was a major stockholder in the company, which now supplies half the world's fertility drugs. But after a 30-year struggle, the family had gained an 86 percent share of the global conglomerate it had founded in 1906. The growing awareness of infertility throughout the 1980s, and the increasing number of couples who aggressively sought treatment, was a tribute to the company's imaginative marketing efforts. By the end of the decade, Serono's U.S. sales were growing at the rate of 30 percent a year.

Serono landed in America during the 1970s, opening its first U.S. subsidiary in Boston with little more than a dozen employees and no sales force. "If there is a model for this company, it is that you start a new geographic area on a grassroots basis," explained Thomas G. Wiggans, president of Serono Laboratories Inc. in 1990. "There's not a large amount of investment. There's a general manager hired and a small operating budget supplied and the orders to grow the business." Serono enjoyed a virtual monopoly on one of its best-selling fertility drugs, but as it tried to expand into new markets it faced daunting competition from some of the largest drug companies in the world. The company also had to overcome the sense of helplessness and fatalism that kept many infertile couples from seeking treatment. It had to sell hope to the hopeless.

In lieu of conventional advertising, Serono created its U.S. market with patient education seminars and medical symposia. This method was cheaper, and infinitely more effective. The demand for raw information among men and women struggling unsuccessfully to conceive a child was so high that the company could charge admission. In 10 years, the firm held 92 major conferences for infertile couples in every large U.S. city—always in partnership with a local chapter of the major national patient support group, Resolve. The chapter chose the subjects and speakers; Serono paid the expenses. The chapter got a percentage of the registration fees. The northern California chapter of Resolve, for example, made $11,000 from its Serono-sponsored symposium.

Serono also conducted up to 65 major professional symposia every year, organized and led by the field's preeminent scientists and physicians. The doctors and nurses paid registration fees and earned continuing-education credits. They rubbed elbows with the scientific celebrities in their field. The company became a dominant presence in the American Fertility Society, which counted 11,000 doctors, nurses, and infertility specialists as its members. It sponsored lecture tours, awarded fellowships, defrayed medical publishing costs, and helped organize international conferences. "We are going to become such good friends with the infertility specialists that they will buy anything we have to sell," one Serono executive said. "We want to become the IBM of infertility."

The oldest fertility drug on the market was clomiphene citrate, sold as Clomid by Merrell Dow Pharmaceuticals or as Serophene by Serono. Doctors initially tried it out as a contraceptive, but they quickly discovered that it had just the opposite effect—it spurred the production of eggs in women and elevated sperm counts in men. It also boosted the chance of producing twins from about one percent to almost eight percent. If it was a total failure as a birth-control measure, it quickly caught the eye of infertility specialists who saw it as a perfect prescription for the 500,000 women who had trouble ovulating. It also quickly earned special treatment from Congress, which routinely exempted foreign shipments of the drug from any import tariffs or duties. By the beginning of the 1990s, there were a half-dozen or more combinations of fertility drugs in use.

When conception clinics held family reunions, every baby was guaranteed a Serono balloon. In its patient meetings and scientific symposia, however, the company religiously avoided the appearance of advertising. It would not allow its sales executives to address the participants from the podium or distribute sales literature. It would not even allow the trade names of its products to be mentioned. By avoiding any overt commercialism, the firm carefully nurtured its credibility with patients and practitioners. It also sought to avoid legal problems with the FDA.

In 10 years of patient conferences, 16,000 prospective parents gave their undivided attention to Serono's basic consumer message: Infertility can be treated. Thousands of doctors and nurses every year were getting an equally powerful company message: Treating infertility can be very profitable.

"With so many Ob/Gyns getting out of obstetrics because they are concerned about the liability issues in that area, they need a means for expanding their practice. Infertility is a beautiful area for them," explained Isabelle Stillger, Serono's vice-president of marketing and sales.

The National Institute of Medicine found that doctors were so leery of malpractice litigation that one in every four family physicians had dropped obstetrics from his or her practice. Some simply refused to deliver babies for lawyers or treat their wives. In a half-dozen states, the cost of malpractice insurance per delivery was higher than the insurance reimbursement rate.

All a doctor had to do, really, was to express an interest; Serono's marketing team would do the rest. "We will bring him through the whole gamut of teaching tools that we have," Stillger said. "We have mechanisms for him to increase his patient volume. We have mechanisms to explain how to teach his patients about infertility. Our representatives are not only working with the physicians, but they spend a tremendous amount of time with the nurses in their offices and the office managers. We have materials for their waiting rooms, videotapes on our products that patients can review while waiting, and all kinds of little pamphlets they can read through.

"We get our new users the most business that we can in terms of expanding their practice." Stillger shook her head. "Well, a lot of them just don't know how to run a practice, you know. We have materials to help them do just that. We had a consultant help us put together a practice development program for these guys."

And it paid. At the beginning of the decade, the company's U.S. sales barely topped $1 million. In vitro fertilization was a laboratory curiosity, and the handful of clinics that performed it had abandoned fertility drugs. Less than a dime of every dollar that an infertile couple spent on conception went to buy fertility drugs. By the decade's end, more than 200,000 women were using fertility drugs. Serono Laboratories was selling $111.6 million worth of its drugs, its U.S. work force had grown to 420 employees, and its production facilities were strained to capacity. The *Boston Business Journal* reported that the Serono subsidiary, now the largest biotechnology company in Massachusetts, was selling its fertility drugs in the U.S. for prices four to five times higher than it charged for the same product in other countries. The company counted 1,355 dispensers of its best-selling fertility hormones—each one a doctor who, in effect, was a salesman for thousands of ampules of the company's products every year.

"In ninety percent of the cases where female infertility is the problem, one of our products will be used," Stillger said.

Serono still had a long way to grow. The congressional Office of Technology Assessment estimated that there were 46,500 doctors treating infertile couples. Only about 1,000 were board-certified reproductive endocrinologists. Most were general practitioners, obstetricians, or gynecologists. Some were urologists and surgeons. Only one in 33 was prescribing Serono products.

There was cause for caution. Pergonal, one of Serono's best-selling drugs, was so powerful that sophisticated athletes routinely used it to conceal the presence of performance-building anabolic steroids. When first introduced, improper monitoring of Pergonal caused the deaths of several women whose ovaries were overstimulated. Their ovaries swelled to grapefruit size and burst, causing massive internal hemorrhaging. More frequent monitoring reduced the risk of hyperstimulation to less than one percent, but increased the cost to about $500 to $1,000 a week. The company still warned of side effects that included abdominal pain, weight gain, enlarged ovaries, and, in one of every five pregnancies, multiple births. Every prescription for Pergonal warned about the odds of producing twins, triplets, and quintuplets. The chances that nature would produce quintuplets and quadruplets were estimated at between 10 million and 40 million to one. Doctors who improperly prescribed Pergonal created a national wave of quints and quads—born, more often than not, premature, with underdeveloped hearts and lungs. Frequently they were dead on delivery.

In 1989, a thirty-year-old steelworker's wife from Warren, Ohio, gave birth to quintuplets conceived under the stimulation of Pergonal injections. Sixteen doctors were in attendance. The babies were two months premature; one infant was stillborn. Doctors said her womb was so crowded that there had been no room along the uterine wall for the baby girl to obtain nourishment through the umbilical cord. In the same year, a woman from Detroit who took Pergonal to get pregnant delivered five baby girls 16 weeks premature. They were the third set of quintuplets born in the Detroit area in 15 months. All were products of Pergonal. In Pittsburgh, the bewildered father of four girls and a boy conceived with the aid of Pergonal and born one minute apart said that to accommodate them all, he would have to convert the master bedroom into a nursery. In Nashville, all but one of Tennessee's first set of quintuplets died within a day of birth. They had been conceived with Pergonal. They were buried in a closed coffin flanked by an honor guard of four teddy bears. The sole survivor spent his first four months in the hospital.

Quints in Peoria. Quints in New Jersey. Quads in Stanford and Chapel Hill. At the Georgetown Hospital Reproduction and Infertility Center in Washington, D.C., only one woman had ever conceived quintuplets. Only one woman there had ever conceived quadruplets. Both conceived with the aid of

Pergonal. Both chose to abort them all. Although it was possible to selectively abort some, but not all, the fetuses a woman carried, the procedure was so difficult that only a few medical centers offered it. Many doctors, troubled by moral qualms, did not tell their patients about the fetal reduction procedure, and many patients, even if they were aware of the option, recoiled from the idea of selecting one fetus over another. The two women at Georgetown later conceived again. One had twins; the other had triplets.

Tens of thousands of couples throughout the world credited Pergonal for their children's births. In the quarter-century that the drug had been on the market, the company had never been directly involved in a lawsuit. To settle a malpractice suit arising from its use of Pergonal, a California fertility clinic agreed to pay as much as $6 million. Mrs. Patti Frustacci and her husband sued the Tyler Medical Clinic after she gave birth to septuplets—four boys and three girls. One was stillborn; three died within 19 days of birth. The survivors had cerebral palsy. The Frustaccis sued the doctor and the clinic, but not the drug company. Her lawyers argued that the doctors did not properly monitor the fertility drugs they had prescribed to her. The clinic argued that she doubled her dose of Pergonal in a misguided effort to up her chances of having children. The clinic admitted no wrongdoing, but, as a trial jury was being chosen, it agreed to pay the couple $450,000 immediately and then an additional monthly payment to each of the three surviving children for the rest of their lives. The insurance company said it was the only claim it had ever settled involving an infertility clinic.

When the settlement was announced, Mrs. Frustacci was again pregnant—this time with twins conceived with the aid of the same Serono fertility drug.

Around the world, Serono was selling its drugs as fast as it could make them. Worldwide, company sales had grown tenfold in 10 years. Company executives were confident that annual sales would double again to top $1 billion by the mid-1990s. Much of the growth was expected to come from the U.S. market. But company executives were already eyeing Eastern Europe and the Soviet Union.

"We want to make sure that when physicians, pharmacists, and nurses think about infertility services, they think about Serono," Stillger said. "From a competitive standpoint, that's the best way to do business. I think we're going to make it a lot more expensive than our competitors think to compete with us."

As Serono's sales continued to soar, company executives worried how they would meet the demand. Traditionally, Serono obtained its key hormones by processing urine from menopausal women. "Frankly," one company executive explained, "it is not a business a lot of people want to get into. You have to collect tons and tons of urine." For years, the company's most reliable supplier had been an order of Catholic nuns. Although the Church formally disapproved of the technology as a means of conception, the order apparently found it an acceptable source of revenue.

To secure its supply, Serono spent $10 million in 1989 to acquire the patent rights to the human genes responsible for the key female fertility hormones. From now on the company would trust its corporate fortunes to genetically engineered bacteria—not to the elderly nuns.

If there would always be an England, it would always look like the village of Bourn: a Cambridgeshire Kodachrome of brick red, pasture green, and casement gray in which thatched cottages and restored farmers' bungalows clustered around the twisted spire of a centuries-old Anglican church. Every house had its name carved in the lintel. Every hedgerow, every garden flower, every gravel pathway stone—like the families who tended the farm fields framing the crossroads community—had its place and kept to it. Silhouettes of ancient tombstones broke the horizon line like crooked teeth. On the rustling wind, hushed voices carried for a hundred yards. Hoofbeats echoed along the main road. The nearest landmark of note was a wooden gibbet marking the site of an eighteenth-century hanging. A pub signpost staked in the center of the one road that snaked between the front yards boldly proclaimed the presence of The Red Lion and Whitbread on tap. A small arrow pointed the way past the churchyard and across a vestigial moat to a sprawling 22-acre Jacobean estate where the De La Warr family, who gave their name to an entire state in America, once held sway. There, in an imposing country manor built in 1602, perfumed by a formal rose garden and flanked by a six-hole golf course, was the Bourn Hall clinic.

The isolated manor house was the oldest and most successful test-tube baby clinic in the world. So many children had started life in its laboratory dishes that the name of the village where it was located—Bourn—no longer sounded coincidental. No infertility center had achieved greater fame.

Yet the dazzling success of its laboratories was not reflected in its business office balance sheets. The clinic rarely, if ever, showed a profit. At the height of its success, Bourn Hall teetered on the brink of bankruptcy. Drained by an ambitious $7 million expansion program, despairing of ever balancing its books, by 1988 the clinic's partners would be prepared to liquidate—victims, in a sense, of Bourn Hall's success.

Since 1980, when a gifted English embryologist and his gynecologist partner converted its stables and haylofts into a premiere medical facility, Bourn Hall had been a Mecca for couples seeking to conceive a child of their own. From India and America they came, from Singapore, Athens, and Abu Dhabi. They trooped through its baronial front door, passed under the ancestral motto inscribed in the archway, "Jour de Ma Vie," and paid more than $3,500 per treatment cycle. In between shots and blood tests, the women would wander the grounds in nightdresses like wraiths. From Iceland, the couples came in tour groups of six or a dozen at a time, their expenses covered by the Icelandic government, which had contracted with the clinic to treat all its infertile citizens. By 1990, 121 Icelanders had made the 2,000-mile pilgrimage to Bourn Hall. Fifty-four babies were born as a result. In total, Bourn Hall and its urban associate clinic in London, the Hallam Medical Centre, were responsible for 8,000 pregnancies. More than 2,500 of them were produced through in vitro fertilization alone.

Many of the villagers weren't sure they approved of the baby factory that had opened in the manor hall, or what to make of the foreign voices in their midst. But the money to be gleaned from this unusual tourist trade helped quiet any moral misgivings. The villagers rented spare rooms to the visitors, cooked them breakfast, or sold them cakes and ale.

"I wasn't sure I thought it was right morally, but I've become accustomed to it," said one retired farmer's wife who occasionally opened her house to paying guests. "If you can't have a child, perhaps it's a safety measure. It's like nature, isn't it? When a horse or a cow gives birth to a bad one, they reject it, don't they? I think it's the same, really. You see the men walking through the village. Most of them look like grandfathers. I don't know what the age limit is, but I can't imagine any of them becoming fathers." She continued: "You can always tell the Arab patients. Their wives walk about a mile behind them. I always want to tell them that they'll have to get closer than that if they want to make a baby.

"Some of the women stay here and never say a word. Some of them can't stop talking and then I try to lend a willing ear. I had one sweet girl from Iceland. She had come here four times. All she ever had for breakfast was a little bit of yogurt. I didn't like to say anything but I wanted to tell her: If you have a decent breakfast, love, you'll get pregnant."

So many children had been created in Bourn Hall's embryo laboratory that when a fraction of them gathered for a kind of family reunion in 1989, there was no building or circus tent large enough to contain them all. The children sprawled in unruly ranks across the lawn on a sultry May Sunday afternoon—more than 660 squalling, giggling, squirming little people, clutching pink, white, and yellow helium-filled balloons. To accommodate them, the clinic built a temporary playpen from 1,000 yards of safety fence. Some Bourn Hall babies were still in prams wheeled by proud parents. Quite a few were old enough to be led by the hand. Some were still specks in an embryo incubator. Three thousand were frozen in its embryo tanks.

At the front of the crowd stood a chubby eleven-year-old named Louise. She wore a pink party frock and held a yellow balloon. At age eleven, she was the oldest of them all—the first human being to be conceived outside the body. Louise Brown was the first child of a British truck driver and his wife.

She grew from an embryo created by Professor Robert G. Edwards and Patrick Steptoe, the pioneers who founded Bourn Hall. Unlike the crowd of children behind her, she was conceived without the aid of any fertility drugs. The two pioneers, working with the mother's natural cycle, retrieved and fertilized a single egg that grew into the little girl. Pioneers Ian Johnston and Alexander Lopata in Australia, following Edwards's example, also conceived their first test-tube babies without fertility drugs.

John and Lesley Brown's six-year-old daughter, Natalie, stood next to Louise, holding two white balloons on a string in her left hand. The sisters shared more than a loving mother and father; Natalie also had been conceived in Bourn Hall's laboratory, nurtured from an embryo cultured by Jacques Cohen.

"There were so many gods at Bourn Hall," Cohen later recalled. "Psychologically, it was very, very intense. There was so much laughter, so much anger and ambition. It was intense because there were so many gods. It was a little bit like Mount Olympus." For a time, in the early years when the clinic stood virtually alone in the world, Cohen had a foothold in the pantheon.

His first glimpse of Bourn Hall never left his memory. He'd answered a help-wanted ad placed by Professor Edwards in a science journal. When the call from Edwards came, Cohen had been out of work for four months. He took the night boat from Holland, then drove the four hours to Bourn in a Honda Civic.

"When I saw the Hall, it flabbergasted me. I was shaking. Edwards was a living legend. It was so far advanced from what I had been doing. I had seen occasional human eggs, I had already frozen human embryos. But still it was a very special thing. Each human embryo was like a new person I had never met. When I went to the Hall, they were already running a thousand cases a year."

Cohen moved to Bourn, but he went alone; his wife refused to leave Holland.

"Edwards worked very hard on my wife. He worked so

hard he made her cry. I had seen her cry very rarely," Cohen would remember. "She knew that I was unemployed. She knew this was my profession and my love. She was not interested in going with me." They divorced. His thickly accented English and Continental clothes became one more curiosity for the villagers to discuss.

He had arrived flushed with ambition and awe; by the end of 1985, he had resigned in disappointment. Five years later, the regret and the yearning were still raw in his voice—like a son still uneasy over the memory of a domineering father. Cohen had wanted to break new ground. He felt held back in his research.

"In actual fact, they wouldn't let me try new techniques. I wanted to do micromanipulation and they wouldn't let me. I wanted to do embryo freezing and they wouldn't let me. Bob Edwards wouldn't let me." Cohen offered excuses for his mentor, but it was clear he didn't really believe them. Edwards, he would say, was under intense public scrutiny and constant attack.

At the clinic's reunion party, Edwards himself recalled the public pressure for the gathered parents and guests: "We were subjected to vast criticism and not a little personal abuse, from professional colleagues and from others whose most frequent cry was that we should not play God, and not interfere with nature." The worldwide headlines hailing the birth of Louise Brown only fanned the criticism. Edwards believed that techniques like embryo freezing and micromanipulation posed too many ethical problems. When Parliament appointed a government panel to report on the new technology, he suspended the most controversial experiments. They had to step carefully, he cautioned Cohen.

Whether or not Cohen actually took the risk of public opposition seriously, he was haunted by the sense of missed opportunities. "It took Edwards one and a half years to say yes to freezing. I mean, he employed me to do embryo freezing and then didn't want to do it. It didn't make sense. So the Australians beat us—but only by a few months. It took them a few years to get a pregnancy with freezing. It took us a month.

When we had permission to do it, it took us only a month."

Edwards did not appreciate his part in Bourn Hall's success, Cohen believed.

"It was already the biggest. It was already the most famous. But, because of us, it then also became the best program in the world," he said.

Cohen quit and moved to London, then to Atlanta, and on to New York. His lab partner at Bourn, Carole Fehilly—one of her generation's most gifted embryologists—married and moved to Canada, where she developed the techniques for performing embryo transplants, creating completely new species of animals by fusing parts of different embryos. Several of Bourn Hall's senior medical staff quit to open their own clinic nearby. But in the clinic's converted Tudor and Victorian stables, where its embryo laboratory and operating theaters were housed, Cohen's imprint lingered. The lab still operated on the lines he established, the technicians there said. The clinic's storage vats still brimmed with embryos he had frozen. "We went through a bit of a trough when Jacques left," said Dr. Michael Macnamee, the clinic's deputy scientific director. "There wasn't the innovation in embryology that Jacques would have provided."

In the years after Cohen resigned, the clinic embraced the innovations he had pushed. In a pamphlet summing up Bourn Hall's first decade, five of the 10 milestones cited in the text involved embryo freezing. In the summer of 1990, Bourn Hall announced to its patients that the clinic was ready to introduce two new micromanipulation procedures designed to improve a patient's chance of becoming pregnant. "This will allow us to achieve two of our long-term aims," the clinic's quarterly bulletin noted: "To increase the pregnancy rate beyond 50 percent while reducing the number of multiple pregnancies." There was no mention of Jacques Cohen, or that, working in a cramped clinic far from the village of Bourn, he had pioneered the procedures on his own.

The snubs no longer seemed to sting. "I am actually very pleased about Bourn Hall lately," Cohen volunteered one August afternoon. "On Thursday I was asked officially by the new owners of Bourn Hall to replace Bob Edwards when he retires. They called me."

He turned them down.

In the summer of 1988, as Bourn Hall quietly prepared to close its doors, the Ares-Serono Group bought the clinic for a rumored $12.6 million. Neither the company nor the clinic's former owners would reveal the exact purchase price. What began as a bucolic private practice devoted to the infertile became a corporate showcase. Only months before it learned Bourn Hall was on the block, Serono purchased the prestigious Hallam Medical Centre in London for an undisclosed sum. The company first tried to buy the Bourn Hall name to use as a trademark for a product line, then acquired the entire property. The company merged the two internationally known conception clinics into the world's largest infertility center. Together they accounted for one-fifth of all the test-tube babies ever conceived.

"The company now has a window on reproductive technologies in a way that we never had before," explained Serono's Thomas Wiggans. "We always had good relationships with clinicians, but, to be blunt, we didn't own them. Now we do."

Serono spent $26 million to turn its new Bourn–Hallam Group into an international training and research center for infertility specialists. London University accredited Bourn Hall as a public research institute authorized to train graduate students. The clinic announced publication of the *Bourn Hall Textbook of In Vitro Fertilization and Assisted Reproduction*. The cost of a five-day Bourn Hall training course was $2,570. The new textbook cost $80. Serono executives had in mind a more long-range return on the company's investment.

"Bourn Hall has one of the highest success rates in the world and we can use it as a training center," said Wiggans. "Now, hopefully we'll send a guy over there who is not using a lot of our product or who is not doing in vitro fertilization at all, and when he comes back, he will." If a doctor couldn't afford the trip, Serono subsidiaries in the United States or the United Kingdom would pay the way. In 1991, Wiggans became managing director of Serono's operations in the United Kingdom.

"There is no overt selling here, but in the end, all the visiting doctors are going to be using Serono products. People will learn to use them here. All Serono's main product lines are infertility-based. Anything that enhances the awareness of infertility helps them," said Macnamee, Bourn Hall's assistant scientific director.

Serono rarely missed an opportunity to protect and expand its market niche. When, for example, British lawmakers considered legislation to restrict experiments on human embryos and impose tighter licensing requirements on infertility clinics, Serono commissioned an opinion poll showing widespread public support for such research. At the height of the heated debate, Serono released its favorable poll results through its allies in Parliament. Some of the bill's leading proponents— distinguished British scientists and doctors—were, unknown to the public, company employees or consultants. When the U.S. Congress passed the Orphan Drug Act, which grants a monopoly to the manufacturer of a rare but essential medical compound, Serono was quick to use the new law to secure exclusive sales rights for one of its fertility products. When the same legislation blocked the company from selling genetically engineered human growth hormone in the United States—potentially worth up to $150 million a year—it lobbied energetically to amend the act.

When the U.S. federal government refused to underwrite infertility research, Serono tried to fill the vacuum. On September 14, 1984, the Eastern Virginia Medical School, home to the Jones Institute, announced it had signed an agreement with Serono that would provide $1.5 million for basic and clinical reproductive research. It was the largest private research grant of its kind. Six years later, the company announced that it had patented the fruits of its sponsored research, all covering a variety of new hormone treatments for infertility.

In one of its first acts as Bourn Hall's new landlord, Serono stepped up the clinic's research program. New laboratories were constructed. Professor Edwards, as the clinic's scientific director, was placed at the head of a team of 16 scientists. The clinic announced that the new team was investigating prenatal diagnosis of embryos to detect cystic fibrosis and other genetic diseases. The clinic also experimented with fetal tissue to regenerate human organs. Its first major research announcement involved a new fertility drug treatment "that doubled the full-term pregnancy success rate."

The research group also confirmed that too much of a fertility hormone could be as harmful as too little. Many test-tube embryos failed to implant because levels of fertility hormones were too high. They also determined that this was the same reason why many human eggs often failed to fertilize in the laboratory. Doctors were advised to fine-tune their dosage levels.

Serono solved Bourn Hall's financial difficulties, only to saddle the clinic with an image problem. "People think we have sullied our hands by becoming involved with a drug company," Michael Macnamee said. "The only reason this clinic is private in the first place is because no one would finance the work publicly."

It was ironic. In the beginning, no public agency or national health-insurance plan would underwrite the clinic because its work was considered too experimental. Macnamee recalled that efforts to secure major support from a private benefactor, for example, were thwarted when Catholic Church authorities instructed the philanthropist in question that any investment in laboratory conception would be immoral. When they finally sought out private patients, they were accused of profiteering. A decade later, when only corporate financing would save the clinic from bankruptcy, they were accused of selling out.

The Bourn Hall and Hallam scientists were quick to defend the integrity of their work. Medical director Peter Brinsden assured patients that "the uniquely special ambience and nature of Bourn Hall is being carefully protected." In deference perhaps to staff sensitivities, the company stayed out of the limelight. Neither Serono's name nor its financial interest in the clinics was mentioned in Bourn–Hallam Group press releases, or in the patient-information kits, or in the course announcements mailed to physicians.

"Bourn Hall has never been a great money-spinner," Macnamee said. "We had an ungainly price structure. Referral letters would get lost. We actually have management accounts now. We can say we are on budget or under budget. No one knew a thing about it before. We haven't made a profit in three years now. The difference is that now no one expects us to."

The new industry's business arrangements were sometimes as experimental as the conception technology itself.

In the United States, laboratory conception was the child of free enterprise. American venture capitalists opened a chain of franchised in vitro fertilization clinics. Another company arranged to inseminate eggs in female volunteers, then flush them into paying customers. In early 1984, the ads appeared in several California community and college newspapers: "Help an infertile woman have a baby. Fertile women, age 20–35, willing to donate an egg. Similar to artificial insemination. No surgery required. Reasonable compensation." It was a baby boom, of sorts. Private investors patented the equipment in the hopes that they could franchise embryo transfer centers in hospitals around the country. Conception technology changed so rapidly that their technique was obsolete before they could field a national sales team. About 15 commercial surrogate-mother services opened to match infertile couples with women willing to bear another's child for a fee. The cost, including the mother's fees, attorney's charges, living expenses, and medical costs, often totaled $40,000. Birth mothers became contract pieceworkers. Ten states passed laws to regulate the practice; two banned it.

Clinics attempting to enhance a couple's ability to conceive also did their best to enhance their ability to pay. As a sub-rosa financial service, many clinics routinely submitted misleading insurance bills to circumvent regulations forbidding payment for in vitro fertilization or other experimental conception procedures. No federal public insurance covered conception procedures. Only a handful of states mandated that private insurance cover laboratory conception. Barely a dozen private insurers sold policies to cover it. Even when reimbursement was available, cost-containment measures placed a cruel cap on a couple's dreams of family. To circumvent insurance regulations, a physician would submit fraudulent bills. He might submit an insurance invoice for uterine sounding in which, when the catheter was removed, several embryos just happened to be left behind. "They just made stuff up," one woman explained. Her embryo transfer was billed as surgery to remove an ovarian cyst. Such billing practices became so widespread that by 1989 insurance companies were forced to adopt special antifraud measures.

Most doctors specializing in conception were reputable, but the absence of federal licensing and reporting requirements made it easy for unscrupulous practitioners to flourish. One metropolitan Washington physician essentially sold false pregnancies. The infertility specialist routinely injected women with a hormone known to cause a positive reading on a pregnancy test even when there was, in fact, no pregnancy. When a fetus failed to develop, he would tell the women they had miscarried, then enroll them in another round of the $5,000 treatments. When he was finally caught, a federal judge fined him $250,000. Former patients filed a dozen multimillion-dollar lawsuits against him. The state medical board moved to revoke his license to practice medicine.

But such aggressive enforcement actions were rarely taken. The Federal Trade Commission started to scrutinize the infertility field only after congressional hearings highlighted its enforcement failures. "The Federal Trade Commission's policy with respect to IVF has been little more than let the buyer beware," said U.S. Representative Ron Wyden, D-Ore., who chaired a congressional investigation of commercial conception clinics. "Success rates are exaggerated and consumers may be grossly misled."

FTC Director William C. MacLeod earnestly assured the congressman that the commission was actively investigating advertising claims.

Wyden, noting that the commission had yet to develop a single case on its own, retorted, "As far as I can tell, you are just reading a bunch of newspaper clippings that the subcommittee sends you."

The ads to which Wyden referred spoke in a soothing whisper: "There's no other perfume quite like it, the smell of a newborn: a milk-scent, cuddle essence. Her skin a kind of new velvet. Toes more wrinkled than cabbage, yet roselike. Tender, soft, totally trusting; a blessing all your own. That dream might still come true for you. New techniques can resolve many fertility problems, including some that were previously considered hopeless. Before you let go of the dream, talk to us." But the dream was all too often a consumer nightmare.

Clinics and private physicians juggled clinical statistics to cast their success rates in the most favorable light. One New Orleans clinic boasted of its 30 percent success rate before it had delivered its first live baby. A Boston clinic spoke of its 236 delivered babies, but the fine print revealed that the clinic had itself never produced a single child; the babies were produced in other cities at clinics operated by the Boston clinic's parent corporation. Some clinics touted statistics based on averaged national results, rather than their own, far lower, success rates. But even the most reputable clinics could not always bring themselves to publish their results openly. Many clinics reported success rates to the American Fertility Society only on the condition that they remain anonymous.

For the couples trying to chose among conception clinics, it was like trying to buy a car when mileage figures, repair records, and gas consumption were closely guarded trade secrets. Left on their own, patients had no way to crack the "code of anonymity" that obscured clinical success rates.

"Every time I have had the opportunity to try to look at somebody's advertising, what we have found is that they are not actually lying," Benjamin Younger, 1989 president of the American Fertility Society, told Wyden's subcommittee. "They just take data and put it into the framework that is most favorable for attracting patients."

When the Fertility Society refused to disclose its own clinic-by-clinic data to Congress by majority vote, it was left to Wyden's subcommittee to develop the first objective consumer's guide to conception clinics. The committee's survey, as thick as a metropolitan telephone directory, was a standardized catalog covering 146 IVF clinics. It made each clinic's track record public for the first time: number of births, types of fertility problems the clinic handled, qualifications of its laboratory personnel, and patient ages. Even under the pressure of a congressional investigation, however, many clinics—including some of the country's largest—refused to volunteer any information.

"There is a resistance to any kind of review of what they do," said congressional investigator D. Ann Murphy. "I don't think the IVF practitioners are any different than most doctors in that sense. They just don't like it. They're on another level altogether from us mortals, and they really don't want to be tampered with in any way.

"We have a responsibility to make sure that the infertile people aren't being exploited. Whether or not we're talking strictly about a legal issue—false and deceptive advertising— is a moot point in my way of thinking. In terms of public education, I don't care if a lawyer reviewed that advertisement and ensured that it's squeaky clean legally. That's not the issue. These doctors and clinics are actually offering a service that is different from selling blenders and microwave ovens and the like. They have an obligation to the patient," Murphy said.

Under Wyden's prodding, the FTC promised to examine infertility clinics more aggressively, including the misrepresentation of success rates, false claims of "guaranteed" success, the use of drugs to trigger false positive pregnancy tests, and the falsification of test reports. The American Fertility Society started framing minimum standards for laboratories that handled sperm and embryos. Legislation to license embryo laboratories was introduced in Congress. If enacted, Wyden's bill would force clinics to report their success rates every year to the Secretary of Health and Human Services. Any violations would result in a $10,000 fine. The Society for Assisted Reproductive Technology, which counted the largest and most successful clinics among its members, voted to expel any clinic that would not make public the detailed statistics behind its success rates.

Long after they were adjourned in 1989, the hearings continued to cause ripples. The letter from Washington arrived at Reproductive Biology Associates in Atlanta almost a year later.

The FTC Bureau of Consumer Protection requested copies of all the clinic's brochures and advertising. The staff investigator wanted the clinic to substantiate a claim made in the clinic consent forms: "Current success rates are approximately 24–26 percent for term pregnancy."

The Federal Trade Commission had already charged two infertility clinics, including one of the largest purveyors of conception services in the United States, with overstating success rates. IVF Australia, which operated clinics in Boston, Long Island, and Port Chester, New York, offering in vitro fertilization, advertised in newspapers and magazines that "more than 28 percent of the couples who complete a cycle of treatment are becoming pregnant," and that "one out of three couples who complete a cycle of treatment is becoming pregnant." In a brochure sent to prospective patients, the company said that "when a patient at an IVF Australia program completes four IVF treatment cycles, the chance of giving birth is about 50 percent." To arrive at such impressive numbers, the company had simply left out a significant number of patients who failed in their attempts to conceive, the FTC charged.

Federal regulators also went after a Boca Raton clinic that boasted in newspaper ads and national magazines: "Our success rate is an impressive 30 percent, well above the national average"—this before the clinic had delivered a single healthy baby. Only four patients had gotten pregnant. The pregnancies had not been confirmed by an ultrasound test.

According to Wyden's survey, most clinics that did a significant number of procedures scored a 6 to 15 percent success rate, though some centers achieved success rates of up to 26 percent. Wyden cautioned that clinics specializing in difficult cases inevitably had lower success rates. To satisfy the FTC query, Joe Massey of RBA wrote back detailing the number of babies born per egg retrieval for each year from 1986 through 1989.

Only in 1986 did the clinic's "take-home baby rate" fall in the range indicated in its consent form. In 1987, the rate was 21.9 percent; in 1988, 23.5 percent; in 1989, 22.9 percent. During the four years, the clinic produced 212 babies for an overall success rate of 23.6 percent—certainly an admirable record that

ranked among the best in the country. It still was short, however, of the "24–26 percent" mentioned in the consent forms.
That, Massey carefully explained in his letter, was because the
clinic took its frozen embryos into account when calculating
its success rates. A frozen embryo might stay in storage for
years before being thawed and implanted in its mother's
womb, but any baby that resulted would swell the success
rate for the year in which it was actually conceived.

"By calculating the ongoing/delivered pregnancy rates per
frozen embryo thawed for each year, the number of deliveries
which can be expected when the remaining frozen embryos
are thawed and replaced can be extrapolated," he wrote. When
that equation was factored into the total, the clinic's overall
"take-home baby rate" reached 26.6 percent.

He hoped that would satisfy the investigators.

Sitting at the head of a corporate conference table, Vicki
Baldwin—lance-thin, with penetrating brown eyes and sharp,
angular cheekbones—was a coil of barely suppressed energy.

As the guiding hand behind IVF Australia Ltd., she had
opened conception clinics in New York City, Boston, Long
Island, and Birmingham, Alabama. She vowed to open a conception clinic in every U.S. city with more than four million
people and looked to the day when IVF Australia would go
public, trading its shares openly on the New York Stock
Exchange.

Baldwin had a more personal reason for her belief in the
franchise. She was herself infertile; she owed her children to
laboratory conception. Not until the thirty-seven-year-old management consultant moved to Australia with her husband, and
came under the care of Carl Wood and Alan Trounson, did
she conceive. Their first son was born in January 1984. She
eventually had three children in all—two sons conceived in
the laboratory, and a daughter conceived naturally.

"I just thought they had a gold mine there," she said. She
also knew Trounson and Wood were so strapped for research
funds that they held bake sales and sold raffle tickets to finance
their experiments. "I started thinking about ways that this

could be packaged to take advantage of the U.S. market and also channel money back to them," she said.

Four months after her first son was born, Baldwin was in New York City to drum up investors. She wrapped the Australians' expertise into a franchise package and persuaded eight venture capital groups to finance the company. The idea was simple: to offer the world's best in vitro fertilization services within a short drive of every infertile couple's home. No longer would people have to fly to Australia, England, or Virginia to get the best care. No other medical frills. No research. Just standardized in vitro fertilization in a one-stop conception shop.

"I really shied away from this clinic idea at first because it sounded a little bit too much like baby-selling. Initially, I wasn't comfortable with the idea of getting money for producing babies," Baldwin said.

In return for their technology and prestige, the Australian scientists received unrestricted research funds channeled through Monash University. The 50 scientists at Trounson's Centre for Early Human Development were supported by about $1.8 million a year, much of it in local government grants. But the research team still depended heavily on patient support. "Our profits have dropped considerably in Australia, so we don't have so much money to put back into the center and research," said Carl Wood.

The two Australian pioneers joined the corporation's medical advisory board. Through their arrangement with IVF Australia, they were guaranteed $1.6 million over the next five years.

"We thought we would be dead before we saw any money," Wood said. "I thought it would fail, but her persistence made it come together. Up to now we had lived without it, but in the future we will have difficulty living without it."

By October 1985, Baldwin had signed a contract with United Hospital in Port Chester, New York. By January 1986, the facility was under construction. On March 27, the first egg retrieval was performed. The first patient became pregnant and the clinic was in business. Three months later, they opened their second conception clinic. In 1989, they opened in Boston. In 1990, they opened on Long Island. The venture had some unusual start-up problems. In 1987, the company's Port Chester clinic mistakenly implanted a Brooklyn couple's embryos in the wrong woman. She later miscarried. Both couples sued. By the end of the decade, the Port Chester clinic's staff of 50 conducted 1,000 laboratory conception attempts every year, with a $6 million annual operating budget and just over $6.7 million in annual revenues. The charge was $7,165, payable in advance, for a full cycle of in vitro fertilization. With an insurance prescription card, the cost dropped to $6,545. To transfer frozen embryos, the clinic charged $3,400. By August 1989, the Port Chester clinic had delivered 403 babies. More than one-quarter of them were twins. Seventy-three women were pregnant. Between them, they were carrying 100 babies.

IVF Australia cast its eye on Chicago. Baldwin hoped to open a dozen clinics in all. To fuel its expansion, the company raised an additional $8 million from several major insurance companies.

Local practitioners reacted to the company's four-color brochures and regional advertising campaigns like corner-grocery-store owners being squeezed out by a slick national chain. IVF Australia became a lightning rod for hostility to the commercialization of conception—in large part because it wrested control from individual doctors and placed it in the hands of a corporate board. Congressional critics cited it as the symbol of everything that was wrong with the growing baby business. The Federal Trade Commission accused IVF Australia of misleading advertising. Medical colleagues scorned its "McDonald's approach" to laboratory conception.

Baldwin and her fellow executives were stunned.

"Medical politics are a lot tougher in the United States," said Wood.

Baldwin chose her words carefully. "This has been a cottage industry," Baldwin said. "We're different. We're not a university. We're not a private physician's office. We are a corporation in partnership, and the corporate practice of medicine is not something that's been embraced with open arms by the medical community in general."

There were hundreds of conception clinics in a dozen countries. There were free-standing private clinics, office-based infertility practices, hospital-based wards, and medical-school affiliates. Some practitioners were board-certified or had doctorates. Others had attended two-day infertility symposia. Some sought the profit in conception to pay for the research that governments and public medical institutes refused to fund. Others hoped to widen the access to conception services by lowering costs, raising success rates, and increasing the number of first-rate clinics. For most, laboratory conception was another medical cash cow.

In the end they all shared one goal. They were trying to turn the business of making babies into a paying proposition.

9

The Spring Thaw

Sharon Wiker wheeled the squat gray embryo tank out from under the table and snapped open the lid. A fog of superchilled liquid nitrogen boiled into the room. She gently lifted a tear-shaped glass ampule wreathed in frost. She wiped away the ice crystals to read the name and date etched on its side. She checked the name against her lab records.

Dana and John Hobart. Dewar tank No. 3. Ampule No. 630. Freezing date: January 19, 1990. "Failed transfer," someone had noted on the storage sheet. The glass tube contained a single frozen four-cell embryo. By the calendar, the embryo was three months old. By its own internal cellular clock, it had been alive barely three days. It was nine o'clock in the morning on April 15, 1990, Easter Sunday.

In all, John and Dana Hobart had four embryos frozen under their name at Reproductive Biology Associates. Before the day was out, Wiker would thaw them all. Their time for resurrection had come. The embryos would emerge from the mouth of the storage vat and pass into the warmth of a human womb. The four embryos would be given a second chance at life. It was a rude awakening.

"Close your eyes," Wiker warned. She plunged the first ampule into a metal pitcher of lukewarm water. There was always a slight chance, she explained, that the ampule would explode.

Under the lab bench in Atlanta, Reproductive Biology Associates stored almost 700 embryos in five Dewar tanks chilled to minus 385 degrees Fahrenheit—more than all U.S. laboratories had contained in 1985. In New York, Cohen had another 700 embryos in storage. The tanks took up about as much space as a lawnmower and a coil of garden hose. If the level of liquid nitrogen should ever drop, an alarm would summon the embryologist on duty; otherwise, there would be no reason to disturb the embryos until their parents called.

By 1990, 27 U.S. clinics had 7,397 frozen embryos in storage. Three clinics were responsible for half the frozen embryos and three-quarters of the reported births in the country. Worldwide, the number of clinics and the embryos they had frozen multiplied fivefold in five years. In Australia, where Baby Zoe—the first child who began life as a deep-frozen embryo—was born in 1984, 22 clinics had stockpiled 6,653 frozen embryos by the end of 1989. There were, by the best guess, another 20,000 frozen embryos in England and Europe; perhaps 40,000 worldwide. Nobody knew exactly.

Human beings were not the only species finding a future in the embryo tanks. Zoologists, alarmed over the rapid extinction of the world's wildlife, were stockpiling embryos from endangered mammals. At the Center for Reproduction of Endangered Wildlife in Cincinnati, reproductive physiologists stored snow leopards, Bengal tigers, rhinos, antelope, and desert cats in suspended animation. Test-tube tigers, cultured from frozen embryos there, would be a staple of future zoos.

By the end of the 1980s, 132 clinics in 18 countries had thawed 18,322 human embryos. The tally was a clinical narrative of life and death. Slightly more than 10,900 embryos survived. They were transferred into 6,440 women. About 738 women became pregnant as a result. At the time Belgian scientists compiled the worldwide figures, 329 babies had been born. At least 220 women were still pregnant. There were 27 sets of twins and an equal number of girls and boys delivered. There were 216 miscarriages. Some of the initial clinical pregnancies never even made it to the point at which a fetal heartbeat could be detected. In all, only 60 of every 100 embryos could be revived successfully; of those embryos that survived freezing, only four of every 100 would result in a child. There were better odds at roulette. At a handful of clinics, however, embryologists like Cohen and Tucker could narrow the odds considerably.

For all their numbers, the space the embryos occupied in both the laboratory and the public mind was small. The human-seed stock for repopulating the entire planet could fit in two of the larger insulated flasks. The embryos were not alive in the accepted sense; nothing could function at the temperature of liquid nitrogen. Neither were they dead. More than half would, when warmed, revive. They were, one bemused policymaker observed, not quite human and not quite furniture. They could be awakened, adopted, or abandoned. They could implant and grow in any woman's womb. They could stay in storage for 2,000 years. For anxious couples and embryologists alike, they were cryptic promises, like words mumbled in a prophecy.

Under the same table in Atlanta, in Dewar tank No. 1 and Dewar No. 5, the clinic kept the five embryos frozen for Bill and Lisa Fagg in August 1989. Five embryos frozen for Susan and David Parr that fall were stored in Dewar No. 2. "Thaw one and two first," the records noted. In Dewar No. 4, two embryos belonging to Lisa and David Boone had been in storage for eight months.

Life had taken a detour around them. It was uncertain when anyone would attempt to revive them. Lisa and Bill Fagg were shopping for baby furniture. After five years on an adoption agency waiting list, they were expecting to take home an adopted newborn child within the month. "I'd take the risk of keeping our embryos frozen in the hope of some new technology that would help them implant," she said.

The Parrs, emotionally exhausted after three failed embryo transfers, were trying to regain their balance. "You get sucked into it and you forget what is normal. I have to let my body regroup," said Susan Parr. "Maybe I am just gun-shy." Three times, she postponed reviving the five embryos in storage. She bought herself a used Alfa Romeo sports car and pointed out that there would be no room in the two-seater for a baby. By coincidence, the letters on the license plate spelled "MAD."

Lisa Boone was nine months pregnant. Her baby was due any day. Lisa Boone was no longer in the clinic's care, but she still liked to visit the nurses there. She liked to let them touch her swelling abdomen. "They never get to see the results of what they do," she said. "They get us to the point of conceiving or not conceiving and then we disappear. They never see us again." It might be a year before the Boones were ready to revive this child's stored siblings.

The shelf life of a frozen embryo was a matter of clinical discretion. One couple had kept three frozen embryos at RBA on hold for four years before thawing them that April. They all survived, and the woman became pregnant. The couple still had three more embryos in storage, and they had no idea when they would revive them. The case was not unusual. No one could agree on how to dispose of the surplus properly. To prevent stockpiling, authorities in Melbourne imposed a five-year limit on the length of time embryos could be stored. They ordered that any unclaimed embryos be put up for adoption. One New Age entrepreneur proposed that all surplus frozen embryos be shrink-wrapped in plastic and sold in gift shops as a novelty item, like pet rocks.

For half a minute, Wiker held the embryo ampule under water and watched intently as the milky ice inside it cleared. Then, with a diamond-tipped glass-cutter, she briskly opened the ampule, suctioned out the embryo, and deposited it in a well of peach-colored sucrose solution—the first of six shallow wells arranged on the lab dish like the hours on a clock face. The shriveled embryo would soak for a few minutes in each of them, slowly swelling to its normal dimensions.

Wiker set the alarm on a white egg timer to time the bath. An energetic Irish jig played on the laboratory boom box. In the incubation chamber, Michael Tucker prepared an embryo for transfer. Tubes of semen spun in the yellow centrifuge. Dr. Joe Massey leaned in the doorway and chatted amiably with another couple waiting to receive their embryos.

Michael Tucker would never be certain what mistake they

had made in November and December, or what they had done since January to restore the clinic's pregnancy rate. "We started from scratch," Tucker said. "We paid attention to detail and we got it right."

During the clinic's winter cycle, Tucker, Wiker, and Graham Wright collected 402 eggs from 57 women. They created 195 embryos. Of 45 women who received embryos, 15 women became pregnant. Three carried twins and one carried triplets. Two women miscarried. The lab team also thawed and transferred embryos for 16 couples. Three women became pregnant, two of them carrying twins. The three embryologists had yet to become friends, but the months of grinding detail work had transformed them into colleagues. Tensions in the laboratory eased, but not before patients began to sense something was amiss. Some couples brought their complaints to Resolve meetings. The clinic, they thought, seemed distracted, its staff members burnt out. At several board meetings, the local Resolve board of directors debated the merits of presenting formal complaints to the clinic. They hesitated. Some of them were still patients there. Did they want to risk angering the doctors who offered them the best chance for a child?

It was hard to arrive at any objective judgment about the clinic's success or failure. Some of the individual cases had become so complicated that they defied analysis. One woman produced 39 eggs, but when they were inseminated with her husband's sperm, they yielded only two embryos. Those fertilized only after Wright performed the PZD operation on the eggs. When donor sperm was added, six more of her eggs fertilized. She received the two embryos conceived with her husband's sperm and two of the four conceived through the donor. Until the ultrasound scan revealed a single fetal heartbeat, she lived with the possibility that she carried in her womb children conceived by two different men. Now she was pregnant with one fetus. It would take genetic tests to determine who really had fathered the child she carried. "It will be up to them to figure out whether or not it was one of the donor embryos that implanted," Wiker said.

She checked the Hobarts' embryo through the microscope. It was too soon to know if the embryo was alive. It would be hours yet before it recovered enough to begin growing normally again. For the time being, Wiker could only guess.

While the Hobarts' first embryo soaked, she pulled their second four-cell embryo from the embryo tank. "These two embryos were frozen when they were fifty-one hours old. These are her best chance at getting pregnant," she said. She held her hand over her eyes and plunged the second ampule into the warm water. "If an embryo survives through to the first sucrose solution, it usually will survive the entire process," she said. "But even though it is alive, the embryo may never go on to start dividing normally again. Usually you know in about three hours."

Wiker set the timer again and waited.

John and Dana Hobart were not due at the clinic for hours yet. They spent the morning at home. Outside in their backyard, so many dogwoods were in bloom that their house seemed to float among the clouds. When the wind caught the falling white petals, it was like a snowstorm. The nights had been unusually cool that spring and the blossoms had lingered a week past their time.

Every morning for five days, an alarm clock had awakened Dana Hobart before dawn—time for the day's first urine test. Every morning, she expected the clinic to schedule the embryo thaw. Every day, it was delayed while the doctors waited for her body to ovulate. Every day, she delivered urine samples to the laboratory so her hormone levels could be measured. Every day, they checked the condition of her ovaries with an ultrasound probe. To avoid the transfer problems that forced the clinic to freeze her embryos in January, Dr. Massey dilated her cervix. Then he sewed a thread through it. By tugging the stitch, he would be able to pull her uterus into position for the embryo transfer.

In most other respects, the transfer of her frozen embryos would be as natural as laboratory conception could make it. This time, the Hobarts would not participate in any clinical trials or untried embryo operations. There would be no steroids for her to take; no fertility drugs. The embryos would be transferred during her normal cycle. At least she had been spared the need for hormone shots to produce extra eggs this time, because they would use the embryos created the previous January. The doctors believed there was a better chance that the embryos would implant if the lining of her uterus was not irritated by drugs. Her emotions, in the past artificially heightened by the extra hormones, were slowly returning to something akin to normal. But physically, she found the process increasingly repugnant.

"I'm getting worse about this stuff, not better," Dana Hobart said. "I just hate being messed with. When I first went in it was no big deal. But now I don't want my ultrasounds. I don't want to be poked. I don't want any kind of pain at all. Before, because I didn't know what to expect, I didn't get too worked up over it. I just went in and did it. I don't really want any discomfort anymore. I'm tired of them sticking these cold wands in places that aren't supposed to have cold wands in them. Everything seems to be more sensitive. Maybe it's just my imagination."

Less than a year had passed since her first attempt at in vitro fertilization, but the months had altered her reflection in the mirror. The lines were deeper around her eyes and mouth. Her hair had lost its gloss and her skin seemed sallow. She compared herself to the other women in the waiting room.

"Last time I went through IVF, it seemed like I was one of the youngest women there. This time I was one of the oldest women in there. The way they sounded . . . They looked young. They sounded young."

While they waited for the thaw to be scheduled, the Hobarts carefully distanced themselves from hope. "I know what the statistics are," said John. "Only sixty percent survive the thawing process." He had talked it over with his barber, who by now was the father of an entire family conceived at the RBA clinic.

"Did Massey do the fertility dance?" his barber wanted to know. The barber insisted gravely that Massey's fertility dance was the key to a successful embryo transfer. No, John would reply, Massey had never danced for them. Maybe he no longer needed to do it.

John and Dana talked. They worried about how much the

laboratory procedures themselves had compounded their inability to conceive a child by increasing the scar tissue around her cervix and uterus. They constantly reassessed their commitment and their stamina. They added up their medical bills. Insurance no longer covered them; so far that year, they had spent $7,200. It would cost another $1,650 to transfer the frozen embryos. They argued about adoption, which could cost another $10,000.

"What else would we spend the money on?" she said.

"Renovations to the kitchen. Buying a car."

"Why do you always change the subject?" she asked him.

"There's a lot of emotional stock invested in this—emotional capital—and it's hard to equate a human being, your own flesh and blood between the two of you, with redoing the kitchen or buying another car," he said. "But at some point you have to weigh all those things. We've got to come to some point here to where we say enough is enough."

"When did you change your mind?" she asked.

"I feel like we're just not getting anywhere with this," he answered. "I like to have frozen embryos, but that's still not going to put them in the cradle."

Once the embryos started to warm, Sharon Wiker was in a race against time and the thermometer.

Before each embryo was frozen, it had been dehydrated with a chemical called propanediol—commonly found in antifreeze—that leached the water from its cells so that no ice crystals would rupture the fragile embryo. As the embryo thawed, however, the chemical that ensured its survival at minus 385 degrees Fahrenheit became progressively more poisonous. At room temperature, it was fatal. To draw the cryoprotectant from the embryo, Wiker bathed the cells in progressively stronger solutions of sugar.

The technicians froze only those embryos that appeared to be developing normally. The age of the embryo and its stage of development before freezing were perhaps the most important factors affecting its survival.

The embryologists could choose from at least four different types of cryoprotectant to protect embryos during freezing.

Each required a different level of skill and timing. Depending on the chemicals involved, the embryos had to be frozen at a different stage of development and had correspondingly different survival rates. There was reason to believe that the younger the embryo, the more likely it would implant. By freezing an embryo earlier in its development, the technicians could triple the number that would survive storage and lead to a successful pregnancy.

The technology changed so rapidly; there was no guarantee that, when it came time to thaw the embryos, the doctors would still be proficient in the precise technique that had been used to freeze them. The hundreds of storage vials in the embryo tank at Epworth Hospital in Melbourne, Australia—the oldest embryo storage facility in the world—were a mosaic of embryos whose lives had been suspended by so many experimental techniques that only one woman, the senior lab manager, could remember how to thaw them all. The clinic doctors had programmed the thawing techniques into a computer just in case she ever quit. At the Illinois Masonic Medical Center, doctors couldn't decide which technique offered the embryos the greatest chance of survival. So they arbitrarily froze half their embryos one way, half the other. At the Hammersmith Hospital in London, the largest single conception clinic in Britain, doctors thought embryo freezing was so unreliable that they refused to offer the procedure. "There is very little prospect for any of these embryos ever doing anything," insisted Hammersmith embryologist Alan Handyside. "You might as well put them down the sink. The chromosomal abnormalities induced by freezing have not really been worked out." The Hammersmith clinic used excess embryos for research or donated them to other infertile couples.

As with everything else in his laboratory, Jacques Cohen had developed his own system for freezing embryos. To store them as early as possible, when their chances of survival were highest, Cohen invented a way to freeze the embryos safely even before they divided once—at a pronuclear stage when they were effectively no more than fertilized eggs. The frozen zygotes resulted in higher pregnancy rates per embryo transfer than did older embryos. There was another advantage: The procedure took place before the mother and father's genetic material merged to form a unique new individual genome— *i.e.*, before conception had occurred legally.

Wiker wanted to count the Hobarts among the clinic's successes. Wiker was herself three months pregnant, and she had a three-year-old at home. Both times she had conceived naturally. She felt an extra obligation to the embryos arrayed in the tank before her. She rarely spoke to the couple whose embryos she tended; they were only names on an index card. But she would do whatever she could to ensure that they became parents.

Scientists weren't sure what the embryo needed in order to implant properly. The wall of the uterus had to be "primed" chemically by the body's hormones to be receptive to the embryo, but they did not understand how. The rise and fall of the hormone levels, as charted on the lab sheets, were their only guides. They had discovered a set of immunosuppressor cells in the human womb that evidently protected the developing embryo from the mother's immune system. When these cells were absent, the pregnancy failed. The embryo itself secreted special proteins within hours of fertilization that might play a role. They suspected that one reason so many sperm were released during intercourse was that they conditioned the womb to paternal antigens—getting it used to the idea of a stranger.

Wiker's timing was critical. She needed to synchronize the age of the embryos with the expectant uterus. The womb was receptive to an embryo transfer only a few days each month. A few hours either way could mean all the difference.

"This is not a clear-cut thaw. We are not precisely sure when she surged," Wiker said. She stared at the chart of hormone levels and gnawed the pen. There were two spikes on the chart that could indicate the moment Dana Hobart's hormone levels had risen. She consulted with Michael Tucker and then used her judgment. She sometimes orchestrated the procedure so that the embryos were back in the womb before anyone knew if the cells were growing normally again.

To time the thaw, Wiker started with the evidence of Dana

Hobart's hormone surge. She first added 25 hours—the usual time between the surge and ovulation. She added another 51 hours, which was the actual age of the embryos when they were frozen. Then, to account for how slowly embryos develop outside the body, she subtracted 12 hours. An embryo lost between six and nine hours of development for each day it spent in a culture dish. Then, to compensate for the time it took the thawed embryos to resume normal development, she added another three hours. Wiker was nervous. She double-checked her numbers.

When Wiker focused the microscope on the Hobarts' first embryo, all she could see was a cluster of wounded cells. The thaw had crumpled the embryo. It looked like an automobile sideswiped in traffic. "It has sheared," she said.

Fluid oozed like blood from the four-cell embryo. It had been damaged, in all likelihood, the moment it reached room temperature in the water bath. As it thawed, the embryo was so fragile that it could be shattered by a brush with an air bubble.

She quickly examined the second embryo. It also had ruptured.

"This one has a big crack in it."

She swore softly and looked more closely. One of its four cells seemed undamaged. Were they dead? Were they alive?

"I'm going to thaw the others," she said. These were the Hobarts' two remaining embryos, slightly older siblings frozen when they were 57 hours old. At that stage, they consisted of six cells each. The Hobarts had started out with five embryos in all created in two laboratory cycles. One had died after the failed transfer in January before it could be safely frozen.

"It's mush," Graham Wright had said. "We'll have to toss it."

No one told Dana and John Hobart. When the couple counted their blessings that Easter morning, they still numbered five. They kept telling each other, "We have five beautiful embryos."

Five became four. Four became two. The frost. The plunge. The sucrose bath. Wiker moved the last two embryos from one droplet to another. They fared no better. "None of them wholly survived," Wiker said, staring grimly through the microscope.

All that survived were fragments.

"We have one-fifth of one. This one is dead. Well, I think it's dead, but we will have to check it just before the transfer. We really won't know whether it survived or not until then. We have one-fourth of this one left. The last one has four cells alive, but it is coming out of its zona membrane. All I can say is that we'll look at them in thirty minutes and see if they survived," Wiker said.

She telephoned the clinic supervisor.

"We have a two-fifths, a one-fourth, and a one-fourth with a fractured zona," she reported. "I'm going to treat them like they are all alive. I think the faster they go back into her body the better."

What should the supervisor tell the Hobarts? What could anyone say? Perhaps the transfer should be canceled now before they left for the clinic.

But Wiker did not want to admit failure yet. "Tell them to come. We will assume that something will survive. It's usually not this difficult," she said. "It usually is more clear-cut."

To gauge the health of the revived embryo, and its chances of implanting successfully, the lab technicians had only the most obvious physical characteristics to guide them. The spherical shape of the cells, the smoothness of the membrane that encapsulated them, the number of fragments floating inside—these were the signs they checked. Cell damage was common after thawing. Even embryos with two or three physical abnormalities still had about a one-in-five chance of implanting successfully.

The Hobarts' four embryos together had contained 20 cells. Only four of those cells survived their reawakening. Freezing had suspended the embryos so early in their human development that their cells still possessed an enormous potential. No biological choices or commitments had yet been made. Each remaining living cell was at the threshold of a mystery. There was in them a power unlike that in any adult human cell. At this stage, each embryonic cell was enough by itself to grow an entire human being. From a single cell could spring the muscle, sinew, heart, and brain of a healthy child.

What the freezing process had accomplished by accident, some embryologists—working with sheep and cattle embryos—did on purpose. When cattle breeders cloned prized livestock, they did no more than reduce a selected embryo to its individual cells. They cut them apart with a razor and, by culturing each cell, coaxed an entire herd from one embryo.

Not all the laboratory's embryo experiments were planned. Through an accident of circumstance, the clinic had reduced each of the Hobarts' embryos to its smallest living component—an individual cell. The cells were a clinical question mark. Would one be enough to engender a child? There had been reports of a very few pregnancies achieved with fragmentary embryos; the clinic had succeeded in this twice. Wiker put the damaged embryos in the incubator. For the Hobarts, there was a remote chance those few surviving cells could ripen into a pregnancy. "Her best chance is to have all four put back in her," Wiker said.

By the time the Hobarts arrived at the clinic just after noon, they had already learned that their best chance might be no chance at all. Dana stood in the hallway outside the laboratory weeping with anger. She had worn a pair of beaded red moccasins—her "fertility shoes"—for luck. John tried to calm her. "Now, try to maintain a positive attitude," he said.

The nurse who escorted them to the laboratory silenced him with a hand on his arm. "It's okay. It's her right," she told him.

Sharon Wiker passed them in the hall. "They wouldn't meet my eyes," she said.

"Well, I have an overwhelming sense of déjà vu," said John Hobart.

He held the door to the transfer room open for his wife. His one quick glance encompassed the video monitor, the transfer table, and the framed photographs of the embryos hanging on the wall. Dana wrapped herself in a white blanket and settled herself on the table. "Oh, it's cold," she said.

Across the threshold in the laboratory, Sharon Wiker sorted

through a stack of compact discs. "Well, what kind of music do these people like?" She settled on the soundtrack from the movie *The Mission*. A choir of churchly voices filled the room.

The monitor came on. The light flickered on their faces in the darkened room. The doctors, embryologists, and the Hobarts all stared at the magnified image of the embryos on the screen. "Are you any good at elementary-school math?" Massey asked the Hobarts. "There is a two-fifths, a one-quarter, and a one-quarter here." Massey peered more closely at the screen. "That one doesn't look too bad," he said almost to himself. "One of them had better work."

More than three-quarters of the embryos that survived the freezing tanks had at least two obvious physical abnormalities. How much damage could an embryo sustain? The doctors had their rules of thumb. Most clinics around the world considered a revived embryo suitable for transfer if its protective zona membrane was still intact. Fifty-eight centers would transfer it if only half of the embryo survived the thaw. Seventeen centers would transfer the revived embryo if a single cell was intact.

"At this stage, one cell can make it," Massey told the Hobarts. "One cell can implant and develop a pregnancy. They can survive. It would have been better, of course, if you had one embryo that had all four of its cells survive. We are hopeful they will stick. We have had only a handful of fragmentary embryos—less than five—that have continued on to a pregnancy. Today is a fertile day," he said in a heartier voice. "All the omens are right today. We need omens around here."

He adjusted the speculum. Sharon Wiker handed him the loaded transfer catheter. The transfer was quick. Dana Hobart, braced for more pain, was surprised and skeptical. "Did they really go in?" she asked.

"In like Flynn," Massey replied. Normally, this would be the moment for him to wish them luck, for them to offer a handshake in return. Wiker would present the photograph of the embryos. There was instead a silence. No one believed the embryos would survive.

Dana sat up on her elbows. "You have to do the dance," she told Massey. "The fertility dance."

No, he didn't think so.

She locked eyes with him. "Is it going to work this time? Guaranteed?"

He looked at her. She had been in his care for two years. He could feel their anger and anguish. He thought of the living fragments he had placed inside her and how slim their chances were of survival. Together, in a windowless room on Easter Sunday, Massey, Wiker, and the Hobarts had reached the limit of what science and medicine alone could accomplish. The cells were on their own. The doctor's bedside manner deserted Massey. Suddenly, he was just a middle-aged man in the dark with a good heart and a medical degree.

So Joe Massey did the fertility dance.

Slowly and sheepishly at first, he flapped his arms and scuffled his feet. The light on his head traveled around the walls as he twirled in a circle. He gained speed. His arms blurred. He burst into a frenetic buck and wing, his hands and feet flying, his head bobbing and weaving. Abruptly, he stopped. The nurses and the lab technicians stared.

He sketched an awkward bow. It would be at least 12 days before any of them would know if they should applaud.

Jacques Cohen prowled the sixth-floor corridor of the Cornell University Medical College with a rubber pipette hose clenched between his teeth and a glass microscalpel in his hand, a medical buccaneer ready to repel skeptics. Manhattan had brightened his wardrobe, if not his mood. He arrived at the lab that morning in a designer's coat of many colors—a bleeding plaid of purple, blue, green, and yellow, worn over a black-and-turquoise shirt, set off at the collar with a cerulean blue bow tie. Inside the hospital, he donned rumpled green scrubs but retained his frown. "They don't believe in me here yet," he said.

After December's debacle, the clinical numbers were running his way again. Between January and March—while construction crews rerouted pipes, ripped out wiring, and tore out the ceiling over the operating room—Cohen and his clinical team retrieved 1,421 eggs from 146 women. They created 836 embryos. One of every five embryos implanted, six times the

national average. One in 10 embryos was abnormal. Fifty-one
women became pregnant, for a clinical pregnancy rate of 39
percent. In a single 33-day stretch, Cohen surgically altered
eggs for 28 couples. Sev Rosenwaks was running out of paper
stars to paste on the laboratory calendar to commemorate each
new pregnancy. The clinic was running at a record pace, with
25 percent more patients than the year before. The embryologists ate dust and turned up the radio to drown out the
jackhammers.

By May, the workmen were gone. Cornell's clinical IVF laboratory, once cramped and crowded, had been transformed
into a spacious duplex encompassing six laboratories, freezing
rooms, and offices—easily one of the largest and most well
equipped embryo labs in the world. Where the clinical embryo
lab previously straddled a major hospital thoroughfare between the maternity wards and a busy surgical arena, it now
was isolated from the rest of New York Hospital by electronically controlled doors, combination locks, and digital alarms.

On this day, Cohen was intent on staying as far from the
clinical lab as possible. Two floors away, he paced restlessly
in Cornell's Embryo and Gamete Research Laboratory. There,
overlooking the walled campus of Rockefeller University along
the East River, Cohen, Henry Malter, and Beth Talansky had
created a research laboratory in their own image. The space
had been gutted and redesigned. Construction crews built in
wraparound desks and marble-topped lab benches. They in-
stalled brand-new laminar flow hoods, cell manipulators, and
incubators. Malter lost no time pasting a new gallery of tabloid
headlines on the freshly painted walls:

"Siamese Twins Born Pregnant."

"Brain Dead Women Used to Grow Babies."

"Grieving Parents Freeze-Dry Baby . . . and Stand Him in
the Corner."

On Cohen's U-shaped desk, someone placed a life-sized
cardboard cut-out of a toddler. "Instant Infant. The Perfect
Baby: Absolutely adorable. Not an ounce of work. Zero chaos.
A real gentleman," its caption read.

Flanking Cohen's office window, there were hung photographs of his two ex-wives and color portraits of human em-

bryos. The $12,000 sculpted black cube of a "NeXT" computer occupied the space under the bookshelves. In an adjacent alcove, Beth Talansky dissected hamster oviducts with a pair of metal tweezers. Each ovary was barely the size of a sesame seed. She neatly spilled the hamster eggs onto a microscope slide. Cohen twiddled impatiently with the micromanipulators. "Eggies!" he sang out to Talansky.

With their hamster eggs and glass needles, Cohen and Talansky were conducting the medical equivalent of a grade-school handwriting exercise—rehearsing a sperm microinjection technique. Only by constant repetition could an embryologist master the precise physical movements the microsurgery demanded. Since New Year's, they had performed the "schlepping" sperm injection procedure with three human patients, but none of the women became pregnant.

Even now, after eight months of retraining lab technicians and persuading doctors to alter their techniques, Cohen was still hard-pressed to find time for experiments. "I haven't done any real research since I got here," he said ruefully.

While the workmen hammered, he laid plans for several experimental trials in the hopes that he could pick up where he had left off in Atlanta. He planned a clinical trial of the sperm microinjection procedure and a series of experiments in which he would grow human embryos in fluids "conditioned" by animal fetal cells. Cohen also wanted to try a kind of electroshock therapy—called electroproration—for sluggish sperm cells. He wanted to attempt a kind of organ transplant for an embryo—a risky microsurgical procedure in which he would actually combine pieces of one human embryo with those from another unrelated embryo. In Atlanta, he had scorned the institutional paperwork. But in New York, which had one of the strictest state laws in the country regulating experiments with human research subjects, he took pains to file all the proper forms with the hospital review boards before beginning his clinical experiments. "I need the protection of the system," he said.

There were false starts. The team abandoned its "schlepping" sperm injection technique. The rate of fertilization was so low that it was clinically useless.

"We never kill any eggs with it, which is remarkable, but we may kill the sperm," Cohen explained.

He tried out the sperm microinjection technique developed by Alan Trounson's team in Melbourne. Out of 37 couples who volunteered, only three became pregnant. Cohen felt certain those three would miscarry.

After months of second thoughts, Cohen was ready to face the failures of the fall. Now that the renovations were finished, he was prepared to start another clinical trial of the embryo-hatching operation, in which he made a hole to release the embryo from its surrounding zona membrane, if only he could persuade another round of patients to volunteer. He still wasn't sure why, after its initial success, the experiment produced so many failures. "It's difficult to get any proof because it's such a black hole. You put them back and you never see them again," he said. But he had a theory.

The clue turned up at a conception clinic in Orlando, Florida, that had tried out Cohen's microsurgery. The doctor placed two altered embryos in a patient's uterus. When the embryologist routinely checked the transfer catheter under the microscope, she spotted the empty sacks of two zona membranes. The force of the transfer had pushed the embryos through the holes made by the embryologist to allow the sperm to enter, like grapes squeezed from their skins. Stripped of their protective membranes, the embryos had no chance of survival. When the doctor was shown the empty membranes, the blood drained from his face. "It was like he had killed them," the embryologist recalled.

Cohen believed that the physicians at Cornell were handling the altered embryos too roughly. "The embryos are so vulnerable. When you squeeze the zona just a little," he said, "you can damage them. It depends on the transfer technique. The hole is an abnormal condition that you have to pamper." If Cohen was correct, that could explain why the hatched embryos failed consistently at Cornell, yet did so well in Atlanta.

At Reproductive Biology Associates, Tucker suspected that they had transfer problems of a different sort. He was seeing too many cases in which the physicians had encountered unexpected difficulties inserting the embryos, as they had with the Hobarts in January. "We had a lot of troubles with the last two IVF cycles where patients would arrive at the clinic who supposedly had no problems," Tucker said. "Then there would be tremendous problems with the transfer. We are a bit more religious about it now." Tucker didn't know what kind of improvement to expect. If the doctor placed the embryos too high in the uterus, they could cause a potentially lethal ectopic pregnancy. If the doctor placed them too low, the embryos could slip out the cervix. If the doctor handled the catheter too roughly, the tube could scrape the uterine wall and become plugged with blood or tissue. "A soft touch during embryo transfer is not something you can quantify," Tucker said.

Joe Massey and Tucker were eager to give the embryo surgery a second chance. Tucker organized another, more rigorous trial of the embryo surgery. The patient criteria were so strict, however, that it could easily be a year before they had enough volunteers. This time, they recruited couples who had no known transfer problems. They tried to reduce the risk even further by using a new, more pliable side-loading catheter to reduce the chance of damaging the embryos when they were injected into the uterus.

"We thought we had invented the embryonic equivalent of sliced bread," Tucker said. "Maybe we are making the holes too big. Maybe we are exposing them to too much sub-optimal culture medium. It is the standard paranoia, but I haven't lost faith in this hatching business," Tucker said.

In Chicago, at the Illinois Masonic Medical Center, doctors had also tried Cohen's embryo surgery. In March, they altered embryos for 15 couples. None of them became pregnant. "We were not impressed," said Dr. Aaron Lifchez, co-director of the IVF clinic there. But their own poor results had shaken their faith in Cohen; for the moment, however, they would blame themselves, not his technique. In the waning weeks of spring, they would conduct another clinical trial, altering embryos for 30 more couples.

Cohen tried to persuade his colleagues at Cornell that another clinical trial of the embryo "hatching" surgery was worth the risk, since the underlying evidence was still compelling. He needed 100 volunteers. He had to rely on the nurses to recruit them, and they were a reluctant sales force. He frowned and chewed on the rubber pipette between his teeth. For the rest of the day, he crouched over the micromanipulator, practicing his microsurgery techniques on hamster eggs. "I am impatient," he said. "I don't feel in control. I am afraid of failure, actually."

Taped to the laboratory wall, one of Malter's newspaper clippings read: NEW GALAXY SHAPED LIKE A HUMAN FETUS . . . AND SCIENTISTS DETECT A HEARTBEAT.

Another announced: MAN GIVES BIRTH.

At 11:30 P.M., Dana Hobart rolled over and closed her eyes. An hour later she was still awake. She walked downstairs and let out the dog. The clock on the kitchen microwave read 12:40 A.M. She sat and wept quietly. At 4 A.M., John Hobart came down in his robe. "Come to bed," he pleaded. "You have to get some sleep. You have to try."

The pregnancy test had been negative; the embryos had not implanted. The blood test had confirmed it that afternoon. She called the clinic from her office for the news. "I was stunned and they were upset." She called her husband. She tried to work, but she couldn't. She left and came home. She couldn't stop the tears; she wept for an hour. When John arrived at the house, he did his best to comfort her. "I kept thinking of what happened to those three beautiful embryos," she said. "When I was driving home, I kept thinking: We're going to be alone for the rest of our lives; we're not going to be able to share our lives with a child," she said. "I kept talking to myself like this, getting myself worse and worse. I drove up in the driveway. The first thing I could think in my mind was, I'm never going to see a little kid run up and say: 'Mommy's home. Mommy's home.' It just really tore me up."

She was tired of trying.

"There's nothing that I can do about this at all. Nothing. I've done everything I can possibly do. I've followed every avenue. I followed all the rules. I did everything the way it was supposed to be done. I am tired of having a broken heart, tired of being upset about this," she said. "I'm tired of my life being so dependent on this one thing. I want something positive to happen."

John Hobart was adamant now that they would adopt. He started making calls to private adoption agencies, if not to find a child, then to save their marriage. When they failed their last pregnancy test, he came home to find his wife sobbing uncontrollably in their bedroom. "I'd never seen her cry so hard. She was saying she was inadequate, that she had killed them." He had to stop this or he would lose his marriage, he believed. "I was so nervous when I called the first adoption attorney," he said. It might take a year or more to find a healthy white baby, he was told. Maybe longer. "The attorney gave us hope, but not false hope." Together they started writing a letter to be placed on file for a birth mother. She had another idea.

"You know you can have a baby," she told him. His sperm could fertilize her eggs, but her womb would not nurture them. Perhaps another woman's uterus would be more hospitable to them. They should use a surrogate mother, she said. "All we need to do is find somebody who will go through it." It would at least be his child. She would love it enough to make it hers, as well. "That way I could have John's baby," she said. "I could look at that little baby and say that's my family. Those are my husband's genes. That would be real special to me. He just doesn't agree with that, though. He doesn't see that at all."

He rejected the idea of a surrogate. There were too many legal complications, and, worse, the woman could change her mind. Lawsuits. Baby M. It would be a nightmare. Adoption would be better. An anonymous adoption would be best. He didn't want to know the mother who gave up her child for adoption. It was one thing for the child to be told about his birth parents as an adult, it was another thing for birth mother and child to be exchanging cards and photographs while the child was growing up. That would make him feel like the child's custodian, he said, not a parent.

He surprised her by saying that he would adopt. She surprised herself; she would try laboratory conception again.

"When it doesn't work, you start thinking of ways to make it work. Suddenly the things you object to aren't quite so objectionable," she said.

Their struggle to conceive had transformed their marriage, strengthening it in unexpected ways, undercutting it in others. Her infertility had changed her sense of her past. It cast a starker light on the circumstances of her own birth and the woman who bore her. By introducing her to the embryos she could not bear herself, it twisted her ties to the future. She felt trapped. If she refused to give up, she would be considered neurotic and egotistical—unfit for motherhood. If she didn't try harder, she would be thought not motivated enough to become pregnant—too selfish and self-centered.

"I just want a baby. Is that so much?"

10

The Body Politic

In a Chicago federal courtroom, two attorneys faced the bench: the gray pinstripe suit on the left, the blue pinstripe suit on the right. Federal District Judge Ann Claire Williams—a small disembodied face framed by enormous gold-hoop earrings and large square eyeglasses—spoke in a quiet, exasperated voice that barely carried to the first row of walnut benches.

Probation violation.

Bail motion.

Denied.

A minute ticked by. The wheels of justice were grinding medium-fine this morning. Judge Williams rested her chin on her right hand and took notes with her left. There was a chrome water carafe, a jar of pencils, a silver letter opener, and scissors at her right; a stack of well-thumbed court papers at her left. On an easel against the wall was a large, yellow paper clock, divided into half-hour segments, that depicted "The Trading Day in the Swiss Franc Pit." The black-and-white eagle of the United States District Court for the Northern District of Illinois spread its wings on the wall over her head.

The court clerk briskly called the second case: "Eight-two–C–4324 Lifchez."

The legal anthill stirred.

Huddled next to the wall at the end of the fourth row on the left, the attorney from the American Civil Liberties Union (ACLU) broke off his conference with co-counsel Lori Andrews from the American Bar Foundation. She stuffed her legal papers into a maroon Ortho-Novum briefcase. Reporters filed into the jury box. The ACLU attorney straightened his red tie and approached the bench. An assistant state attorney general stepped forward. The father of an unborn fetus named Baby Scholberg, for the purposes of legal combat, joined them. The judge examined the papers in front of her.

Before hearing another day's testimony on insider trading at the Chicago Commodities Exchange, Judge Williams was going to settle the right of thousands of women in one of the country's most heavily populated states to conceive children with the most advanced medical assistance available. For the first time, a federal court would rule directly on the right of men and women to pursue the high technology of conception and pregnancy.

Lifchez—actually Dr. Aaron Lifchez, the infertility specialist who eight years before had filed the lawsuit that led to the midmorning legal drama—was nowhere to be seen. He was out jogging.

Aaron Lifchez's lawsuit was almost as old as the first American test-tube baby. It had been a slow, stately struggle over the beginnings of human life between doctors and legislators in the heartland. The lawsuit had languished for so long on a crowded court docket that even Lifchez had largely forgotten about it. The athletic, silver-haired director of IVF Illinois at the Illinois Masonic Medical Center had filed his class-action lawsuit in 1982. "We were deposed and redeposed. The case dragged on and on and on," he said.

At issue was one of the strictest abortion laws in the nation, the first state law to deal directly with in vitro fertilization. Under the Illinois law, an unborn child was a legal person entitled to the right to life from the moment of conception. A one-sentence provision of the law restricted research into human reproduction and the practice of laboratory conception: "No person shall sell or experiment upon a fetus produced by the fertilization of a human ovum by a human sperm unless

experimentation is therapeutic to the fetus thereby produced."
Twenty-four other states had similar laws. Six states banned
embryo experiments entirely. In states without formal restrictions, an election-year threat from a zealous local prosecutor
was often enough to block research designed to improve a
couple's chances of conception.

In Illinois, any experiment not intended for the therapeutic
benefit of an embryo or fetus was a crime. The law called into
question the practice of even the most routine laboratory conception procedures and prenatal testing techniques. Who was
to say what was therapeutic for any individual embryo? During
routine in vitro fertilization, many embryos might be sacrificed
to achieve a single pregnancy. On average, four of every 10
embryos placed in cold storage died when brought back to
body temperature. Sperm injection techniques might fertilize
a woman's eggs successfully in some cases, but produce abnormal embryos in others. Microsurgery exposed some embryos to the ravaging cells of the host mother's immune
system. Genetic tests kept all but the healthiest embryos from
their place in the womb. Had those embryos been helped or
harmed? Additional problems could arise from any medication
or procedure designed to help a pregnant woman. The legislature had separated the interests of the embryo and the fetus
from the woman who carried it, yet without offering any guidance. Doctors had to set their own limits, with no way to know
when—or if—they crossed the line into criminality.

What set apart the Illinois law was not its broad condem-
nation of any experimental intervention into the beginnings of
human life, or that it expressly linked abortion and laboratory
conception. It was that state legal officials, who were sworn
to uphold it, had promised never to enforce it. To a surprising
degree, doctors and infertility specialists in Illinois simply ignored it.

While his lawsuit wound its way to the top of the docket,
Lifchez and his colleagues Yuri Verlinsky and Charles Strom
ran one of the world's most advanced embryo laboratories.
Thousands of times a year, they performed conception procedures that could be considered illegal under any reasonable
interpretation of the state law. Their private, for-profit clinic

at the Illinois Masonic Medical Center was one of a half-dozen infertility clinics in Chicago offering with apparent impunity the most experimental conception procedures available. None of them conducted as many embryo experiments as the clinic Lifchez and Verlinsky managed, but the doctors all skated on the same thin ice—their individual clinical judgment.

Yuri Verlinsky was happy enough to split legal hairs. The experiments he conducted, such as embryo biopsy and polar body diagnosis, could be considered illegal under the state law because the doctors would transfer only healthy, desirable embryos to the womb, freezing and storing any abnormal or defective embryos. "The law said we could do diagnosis, not research. So we do it for the embryo, not for the mother. So it is legal," said Verlinsky cheerfully. The state law explicitly covered the developing embryo from the moment of conception, but Verlinsky and Strom argued that their work was exempt, anyway.

"The legislation depends on definitions and semantics," Strom said. "That legislation was a ban on embryo research. According to our interpretation of the law, we don't work on embryos. We work on pre-embryos. That is the hook we hung our hat on."

The distinction was disingenuous at best. Even among fellow scientists, it was acknowledged as an evasive term. The distinguished British science journal *Nature* urged that, as a synonym for a fertilized human ovum not yet implanted in a uterus, the word *pre-embryo* be banned. "Put simply, this usage is a cop-out, a way of pretending that the public conflict about IVF and other innovations in human embryology can be made to go away by means of an appropriate nomenclature," the journal editorialized.

"As long as we felt that all of these things were directed at enhancing pregnancy rates, we never really took the time to decide whether we were in violation of the law or not in violation of the law," Lifchez said. "Enough people were doing them so it wasn't a consideration, so that law for us has never been an impediment. It was just sort of a de facto accomplished thing."

Other Illinois infertility specialists, however, adopted new techniques only after their value had been proven in other states or other countries, assuming there was safety in numbers. Verlinsky was wary of any accusation that he might be destroying human life. As a safeguard, Verlinsky and Strom never threw away an abnormal embryo. They preserved them all in the limbo of liquid nitrogen, where, if the parents never objected, the cells could stay until the law and the men who enacted it were dust.

Public experiments were banned; private experiments flourished. Doctors made their own law in the laboratory while lawyers, drawn increasingly into the high-tech family planning process, dictated research and treatment policies by default.

Many people were suspicious of government efforts to regulate or intervene in reproduction; the creation of a family was too important to be left in the jurisdiction of bureaucrats. But they were equally reluctant to leave such life-and-death decisions solely to laboratory scientists and doctors. When it came to human reproduction, medical ethics was almost always in direct conflict with scientific curiosity.

Attempts to redefine the beginnings of human life were so divisive that legislators and religious leaders were neither willing nor able to solve the moral and ethical conundrums posed by new forms of conception. Three U.S. Presidents sidestepped the issues as adroitly as possible, as did six successive secretaries of the U.S. Department of Health and Human Services. The only congressional commission authorized to review the ethics of artificial conception was so deadlocked over abortion that, after nearly two years of bickering over staff appointments, its enabling legislation expired in 1990 without the six senators and six representatives on the commission having ever considered a single biomedical or ethical issue. A dozen bills to monitor, fund, or regulate the new reproductive techniques were introduced, and died. Conservative congressmen argued that conception was a matter better left to state and local governments. Many state bills on reproduction were often thinly veiled attempts to buttress anti-abortion statutes. Piecemeal legislation spread the confusion across state and national borders.

Despite its rapid advance, the technology itself should have contained few surprises. After the birth of the first test-tube baby in 1978, medical experts, thoughtful legal authorities, and federal ethics panels wasted no time in outlining the permutations of parenthood made possible by laboratory conception. Despite the advance warning, the technology evolved in a legal void. The legal status of an embryo, the rights of parents, the obligations of clinics, and the rights of individuals to gain access to services were not systematically addressed. During a decade when family values were enshrined in a conservative White House, this new nuclear family was not a fit subject for rational political discussion. Instead, the problems of laboratory conception would be resolved in a kind of national domestic free-for-all.

"Everybody has an opinion either based on preconceived notions, their own family relationships, or religious guidelines, about how families should be created and what sorts of decision-making powers parents should have over their potential children," said Lori Andrews of the American Bar Foundation. "People have very gut feelings about what should happen. I don't expect legislatures to ever produce very coherent laws on this subject."

Judges like Ann Claire Williams in Chicago became the arbiters of the confusion created by science and conflicting values, ruling independently and often in direct contradiction of one another. Each new courtroom drama broadened the debate over private conception and public control. Are embryos children or property? Should frozen embryos have inheritance rights? Should a woman's womb be for hire? Who is really the mother of this child? The father? Couples using modern reproductive technologies quickly discovered that they should consult a lawyer as well as a doctor in order to have a child. In the absence of any clear congressional guidance, couples pursued legislation by litigation. What surfaced in court as matters of contract law or divorce codes often turned preconceptions about parenthood and childbearing upside down. Conception clinics and infertile couples were on a collision course with new laws designed to curtail abortion. One Missouri abortion statute appeared to grant legal rights to all hu-

man eggs fertilized in a petri dish and make illegal the disposal
of any excess embryos. And the one legal ruling that provided
a framework for reproductive rights—Roe v. Wade—had come
under increasing fire as the Supreme Court and the nation
grappled with the question of abortion.

In Andrews's office, the unanswered questions of conception
technology took physical form. From the bookshelves lining
three walls, a cascade of legal briefs, rulings, law review articles, books, transcripts of expert testimony, and magazine
pieces spilled across her desk and pooled onto the floor, covering every inch of the office carpet. "The embryo used to just
make its presence felt by expanding out into the woman's
abdomen," Andrews said. "Now we can peer in through ultrasound, amniocentesis, and embryo biopsy. We know about
the developing embryos in different ways. Once you identify
the gender, you humanize it in ways that weren't possible
before. What more independent entity could you have than
these embryos that are totally outside of the woman's body in
these laboratory dishes? Is an embryo property? One judge
ruled for that. Is it a person? One judge ruled for that. Is it
just an entity subject to the parents' constitutional rights? Another judge ruled for that." Troubling legal dilemmas were
scattered through adoption law, divorce codes, inheritance
statutes, product liability ordinances, negligence standards,
and patent law. They often hinged on the status of the embryo
itself.

"If an embryo is to be treated by the law as a thing, it could
obviously be owned. If, however, an embryo is treated as a
person, it cannot be owned. If it is to be treated as a person,
how are such disputes to be resolved?" said Lord Meston, an
expert on family law in the British House of Lords, during the
1990 debate over embryo legislation. "I do not envy the court
which has to decide what is or may be in the best interest of
an embryo, particularly if the choice is between being implanted or not being implanted."

When a surrogate mother in Santa Ana, California, bearing
a couple's test-tube baby sued for custody of the infant developing in her womb, she was asking a Superior Court judge
for more than child support. She sought to redefine parent-

hood. Unlike the surrogate mother in the celebrated Baby M case, vocational nurse Anna Johnson, twenty-nine, had no genetic tie to the child growing inside her. She had, for a fee of $10,000, agreed to serve as the living incubator for three embryos created with sperm and egg provided by an infertile couple named Mark and Crispina Calvert. One embryo survived and implanted. Johnson sought custody of the child and financial support because, she said, the genetic mother and father were late with payments and were indifferent when the pregnancy forced the surrogate mother to be hospitalized. The woman bearing the unborn child sued its biological parents for custody, child support, and emotional damages. Johnson, appearing on ABC's "Good Morning America," maintained that she had biological and maternal bonds with the fetus, even if she lacked a genetic connection. She said that "the baby, while it's growing inside me, has my cells and my blood nurturing this child, maintaining its life."

The Calverts, in turn, charged that their unborn baby boy was being held hostage. California law presumed that the birth mother was the legal parent of a child, but legislators had not anticipated such collaborative contract pregnancies. When the six-pound, 10-ounce baby boy was born, hospital authorities didn't know how to fill in the birth certificate.

Faced with the same sort of custody puzzle that confronted King Solomon, Orange County Superior Court Judge Richard N. Parslow, Jr., declined to cut the child before him in half. "I can tell you right now, it is not my intention to 'split this baby' in an emotional sense and give him two mothers," Judge Parslow said when he announced his ruling on October 29, 1990. He ruled that, under California law, Anna Johnson had no parental right to the child she carried for nine months in her womb. The child's genetic parents will have permanent custody of the boy, unless his decision is reversed by a higher court.

Alan Trounson set the biological precedent for such pregnancies in 1984 when he successfully implanted an embryo created by one man and woman in a second woman's womb. In the years that followed, physicians reported a small but growing business in which couples hired women to bear their genetic embryos—what medical and adoption experts call "gestational surrogacy." Where once an affluent couple would hire a wet nurse to breast-feed their newborn, they were now hiring women to bear their biological child. One South American couple hired two women to bring an entire family of embryos to term. The first woman gave birth to two boys and a girl; then 10 days later, the second woman gave birth to another boy. None of the children was genetically related to the women who gave birth to them. The women were paid $10,000 each for their maternal labor. The Center for Surrogate Parenting in Los Angeles reported 80 such births, compared to some 4,000 children born through more conventional surrogate mother arrangements in which a woman agreed to have one of her own eggs inseminated for the benefit of another couple.

As of fall 1990, the appeals courts had not resolved the plight of Anna Johnson, but her case further reinforced the idea of a woman as a kind of fetal container. Advanced conception technology had unraveled the biological ties that bind, turning mother and developing child into patients who could be treated separately. The Supreme Court defined the fetus in terms of its ability to survive independently, aided by increasingly heroic medical measures. The moment of fetal viability seemed fixed between 24 and 28 weeks—the time a fetus's lungs were sufficiently developed enough so that it could breathe adequately. But the ability to manipulate the human embryo, like experimental operations on fetuses still in the womb, helped fuel the public impression that medical technology would give doctors the power to save any unborn fetus. "Technology is driving the cult of the fetus: everything that treats the fetus, the egg, the embryo as a patient. Attention ends up focused on the fertilized eggs in the laboratory, not on the woman who produced them," said Professor Lucinda M. Finley, an authority on reproductive health issues at the State University of New York in Buffalo.

Mother and developing fetus became courtroom rivals. Medical advances in the ability to image, test, and treat a fetus changed the legal balance of power between the pregnant woman and the developing infant inside her. Many women were willing to sacrifice their own life to save the life of their child, but now that choice was being taken away from them. To preserve the life of a developing fetus, courts in Colorado, Illinois, and Georgia ordered pregnant women to undergo caesarean section surgery against their will. In one extreme example, a federal judge in Washington, D.C., ordered a pregnant woman dying of leukemia to undergo caesarean surgery—even though her husband, her family, and her physicians were convinced the operation would kill her. There also was a strong possibility that the resulting baby would be born with cerebral palsy, neurological defects, deafness, and blindness. The woman's objections were overridden in a judicial hearing held over a speakerphone as she was wheeled into the operating room. The American Medical Association reported her last words on the subject: "I don't want it. I don't want it." The state, the judge later noted, had an obligation to protect the "potentiality of human life." The mother died, as did her 26-week-old fetus. The court extended its condolences.

The case lived on. In a later appeal, a court-appointed attorney for the fetus insisted on its right to life. Uncertain of what he was hearing, Judge Frank Schweib twice asked if the attorney was "urging this court to find that you can handcuff a woman to a bed and force her to give birth?"

The attorney for the fetus did not hesitate. "Yes," he said.

It was not clear how far criminal justice officials would go in using the threat of arrest and jail to control a pregnant woman's behavior. Women who use narcotics, especially cocaine, are more likely to give birth to children with a substantially greater risk of physical and neurological defects. To curtail a substance-abuse problem that affected more than 300,000 babies born each year, prosecutors came up with novel interpretations of child-abuse statutes and drug distribution laws. To curb illegal drug use, prosecutors in a half-dozen states arrested women for distributing drugs to minors—their addicted newborn babies. The crime was to pass the drug through the umbilical cord that linked mother and child. One Texas teen-ager was indicted for possession of the cocaine found in the liver of her stillborn baby. Other women were charged long enough for all their children to be placed in foster care. South Carolina authorities took one woman straight from the delivery room to jail, still bleeding from her labor. Increasingly, they were not willing to wait until the moment of birth. One expectant mother was placed under house arrest for possession of drugs and kept in custody for the remaining two and a half months of her pregnancy. One pregnant woman who went to an emergency room after her husband had beaten her severely was arrested for child abuse instead, because she had, in the view of the admitting physicians, consumed too much alcohol during pregnancy. She was put under a court order to curtail her drinking until her child was born. At least one woman was arrested for simply failing to follow medical advice.

The interests of the embryo were increasingly pitted against the well-being of the woman who carried it. In 1983, for example, a Boston district attorney issued an opinion that a Massachusetts fetal-research law allowed in vitro fertilization only if all of the viable embryos were implanted in women. The same year, an Illinois federal court let stand a similar opinion by that state's attorney general. Doctors who routinely froze human embryos in Atlanta risked arrest and criminal prosecution if they performed the same procedure in Boston or Chicago. It did not matter that the women who received multiple embryos faced greater risk of losing their pregnancy, or that the resulting children faced a higher risk of birth defects, health problems, or early death. In contrast, an English physician who returned more than three embryos would lose his license.

Some legal experts argued that laboratory conception had already provided the means to resolve any conflicts between the embryo and the expectant mother. They suggested that any pregnant woman who sought an abortion should instead be required to undergo an embryo transfer. The embryo could be flushed from her womb to be adopted by another couple, or placed in cold storage. The procedure would guarantee an embryo's right to life, and would preserve at least an illusion of a woman's reproductive autonomy.

But the status of the embryo itself was still an open question.

When did an individual's life begin? Legislators, legal authorities, and medical experts tried to define the beginning of
human life for the purposes of abortion statutes and patent
law. Confident that technology would move the threshold of
survival ever earlier, state officials reassessed the earliest beginnings of a pregnancy to fix the moment when life begins.
They sought a medical and technical anchor for a question of
faith in which neither science nor religion had achieved
consensus.

As a matter of doctrine, 920 million Roman Catholics, like
the members of many conservative Protestant denominations,
believe that life begins at conception. "The Church cannot fail
to emphasize the need to safeguard the life and integrity of
the human embryo and fetus," said Pope John Paul II. For the
world's 860 million followers of Islam, however, life does not
begin until 40 days after conception. The world's 300 million
Buddhists, who count reincarnation among their religious beliefs, do not consider that life has entered a fetus until it has
developed a face and brain. In the traditional tenets of the
Jewish faith, a child's life is not considered separate from its
mother's until its head emerges from the womb. Many pas-
sages in the Bible and the Talmud refer to human life in the
womb without asserting precisely when the individual human
comes into being. Aristotle believed that it took 40 days to
form a male, 90 days to form a female. St. Thomas Aquinas
believed a developing fetus acquired a soul only after its first
40 days. If, in its first few weeks of development, an embryo
did not seem fully human, the priests of the Greek Orthodox
Church would answer that no one—fetus, child, or church
elder—was fully human until he or she had achieved union
with God.

In their search for legal certainty, legislators and judges pondered the merger of genetic material within the fertilized egg.
They looked for the meaning in the moment of implantation
and the formation of an embryo's primitive neural streak. "You
know, nobody ever cared about the status of the embryo before
in vitro fertilization," said Carl Wood.

When Lifchez first brought suit, the Illinois abortion law
defined human embryos as legal human beings. It appointed

the infertility specialists who created the embryos their legal guardians. If any harm came to the embryo while in the doctor's care, the physician and lab technicians could be prosecuted for child abuse. If an embryo was destroyed, the laboratory technicians could even be charged with homicide. The wording of the provision kept Lifchez from offering in vitro fertilization to his infertile patients. He wanted the entire section declared unconstitutional and the state enjoined from enforcing it.

"Eventually I was told by the attorneys who represented us that they had been told—off the record—that the state's attorney would not file suit or prosecute anyone involved in IVF. With that assurance, IVF programs flourished. One started and soon two more started. The appeal was never resolved," he said. In 1985, the state legislature amended the act to permit clinical in vitro fertilization. The prohibition on research remained. Again the governor vetoed the bill. Again the legislators overrode his objections. As long as the state abortion law was on the books, infertility specialists worried that it was only a matter of time before the legal pendulum caught them on the backswing. "As long as that law was on the books, some conservative element could come into power and begin to enforce it," Lifchez said.

His lawsuit languished in the federal district court system—forgotten, but not gone.

The politics of abortion had shaped the practice of laboratory conception for more than a decade, paralyzing efforts to evaluate the safety of the new conception techniques and the health of the children they produced. The abortion debate overwhelmed scientific considerations and blocked virtually any research effort to investigate the beginnings of human life and "the products of conception."

"The only area in our national life where science is suppressed is, I believe, in the beginning and earliest stages of human life," said Dr. John C. Fletcher, a professor of biomedical ethics and religious studies at the University of Virginia, at a gathering of the National Institute of Medicine.

Kenneth Ryan of the Harvard Medical School concurred: "There is practically no area of science that engenders as much controversy or moral conflict as that related to human reproduction."

As the century's last decade began, federal public-health officials and anti-abortion activists showed no signs of relenting. When Congresswomen Pat Schroeder, D-Colo., and Olympia Snow, R-Mich., introduced legislation to appropriate $77 million for birth control and infertility research, the National Right to Life Committee fought the bill because it would allow scientists to use human embryos as "guinea pigs." In the same year, the National Institute of Child Health and Human Development, established in part to assure "the birth of wanted babies through studies on human fertility and infertility," moved to create six clinical research centers to study patients receiving treatment for infertility. Its plan specifically ruled out any research on medically assisted conception techniques such as in vitro fertilization or GIFT. When a group of congressional Democrats and Republicans together urged an end to the federal ban on conception research, their bipartisan report was ignored. Candidates for senior federal scientific and public-health posts were appointed based, in part, on their beliefs concerning abortion. Finally, Representative Henry Waxman, D-Calif., introduced legislation to prohibit the secretary of health and human services from withholding government funding for any research that had been approved by routine scientific and ethical review committees, unless he appointed a special panel that also agreed the research was unethical. If the bill was enacted, the government's most senior health official would no longer be able to block research based solely on his own moral judgment. Federal health officials vowed the President would simply veto the legislation. While the Waxman bill was being debated, Congress allowed the legislation authorizing its biomedical advisory board to expire. The congressional board, meant to review a range of controversial medical research, became officially defunct in September 1990. "For the first time in twenty years, the federal government has no duly constituted, publicly accountable biomedical advisory board," said Alexander Capron, the board's executive director. "It is too hot for the federal government to handle."

In an act of exasperation, senior officials of the American Fertility Society and the American College of Obstetricians and Gynecologists in January 1991 moved to establish a private advisory board to set ethical standards for research involving human embryos, fertilization outside the womb, or fetal tissue. "Research on fetal tissue and reproductive technologies is going on in this country and will continue with or without government regulation," said Kenneth Ryan, chairman of obstetrics at the Harvard Medical School. The 15-member National Advisory Board of Ethics in Reproduction would provide the research guidelines that federal and congressional officials had been unwilling to discuss. Anti-abortionists quickly denounced the proposed private ethics board as "a tiny elite clique."

The political stalemate owed its origins to a question of safety that arose years before the first test-tube baby was born. In 1973—the year researchers in Australia first made a woman pregnant with an embryo conceived in a laboratory—a researcher in Nashville, Tennessee, was already worried about the health of the children who one day would be conceived outside the womb. Within weeks, the Australian pregnancy miscarried. Scientists suspected the embryo was abnormal. And, in Nashville, Dr. Pierre Soupart of Vanderbilt University wrote to the National Institutes of Health to propose that he determine whether laboratory embryos were genetically flawed. His proposal triggered a political backlash that would make it almost impossible for him or any other U.S. scientist to lay the questions systematically to rest. The real issue was not safety; it was life—and who controls it.

When his proposal became public, the response was immediate and hostile. Religious and right-to-life groups mailed more than 30,000 letters to the board protesting the idea of creating human embryos for research. Opposition ran deep even in the medical community. Despite the controversy, however, the board at Health, Education, and Welfare, which oversaw the NIH, noted in its final report that its expert witnesses agreed "that there has been insufficient controlled animal research designed to determine the long-range effects of in vitro fertilization and embryo transfer . . . A broad prohibition of research involving human in vitro fertilization is neither justified nor wise."

The board approved Soupart's proposal and passed it on to HEW Secretary Joseph Califano. He took no action on it. In 1979, Patricia Harris, who succeeded him, refused to appoint new members to the board. In 1980, the board ceased to exist. Succeeding secretaries had the authority to waive the criteria for ethically acceptable IVF research, in part by reviving the board to approve the waiver. No secretary exercised that authority in part because, in the words of one Reagan administration official, "to take no action will avoid controversy." With no board to condone it, no federal research on human embryos could be approved, and, as the decade passed, the federal government refused to fund any work on human fertilization or embryos. When Soupart died, his proposal had never been formally accepted or rejected. The ban on public funding was unofficial but effective.

"Consequently, questions surrounding the interaction of sperm and egg, fundamental to an understanding of conception and contraception, remain largely uninvestigated. In addition, research into the efficacy of some infertility treatments, such as IVF and gamete intrafallopian transfer, is largely uninvestigated and lies outside the sphere of federal funding and peer review," concluded a team of congressional analysts led by Gary B. Ellis at the U.S. Office of Technology Assessment. "The effect of this moratorium on federal funding of IVF research has been to eliminate the most direct line of authority by which the federal government can influence the development of both embryo research and infertility treatment so as to avoid unacceptable practices or inappropriate uses."

Pro-life groups like the National Right to Life Committee said their concerns about research went well beyond abortion itself to encompass the sanctity of human life. They opposed research on laboratory conception because they believed that fertilized human eggs were human beings who should not be subject to experimentation without the strictest regulation and oversight. They said the dismal success rates of in vitro fertilization made it an unacceptable alternative to natural conception. They were troubled by the practice of creating more embryos than the womb could safely hold. Still, they did not hesitate to block any effort to regulate embryo experiments that would ensure that human embryos were treated with proper respect. They did not hesitate to block federal funds for research to improve the success rates they found so disheartening. If any pro-life activists were troubled by the contradictions, they declined to acknowledge them publicly. This was not a debate founded on reason or rule of law; it was a clash of conscience.

"The federal government is guilty of gross irresponsibility and negligence, no question," said Gary Hodgen at the Jones Institute in Norfolk. "It is true of all the administrations and Congresses that served during this era. Even the people that think in vitro fertilization should not have been undertaken would surely have to admit that forcing a state of non-involvement, of non-consideration, non-debate, non-discussion, to not even develop the issue for examination, let alone what the decision might be, has to be in itself irresponsible.

"So, as though the government didn't exist, this whole army of people working different areas have produced a whole new medical technology. And it evolved without government," he said.

Hodgen himself also was a casualty of the federal politics of conception. When the National Institutes of Health ethics board tendered its final report, he was chief of the NIH pregnancy research branch, a leading light in the federal effort to plumb the mysteries of human reproduction. Hodgen directed his energies at seeking ways to safely diagnose and correct genetic abnormalities in human embryos, with the hope of one day discovering methods to correct birth defects. He saw his work as an opportunity to improve the survival of human embryos. Pro-life activists said it would pave the way to their greater destruction. They argued that embryo diagnosis techniques, when perfected, would lead to more abortions.

To avoid confrontations with NIH officials or Congress, Hodgen confined his research to laboratory animals. Privately, he chafed at restrictions that kept him from translating his findings into clinical practices that could treat human infertility. He soon ran into trouble. First his superiors downplayed his research in their annual reports, then tried to omit all mention of it. They forbade him to discuss it in public. Hodgen dutifully toed the political line, but finally, out of mounting frustration, he resigned and joined the Jones clinic in Norfolk. Many of his federal co-workers moved with him. In one stroke, the Eastern Virginia Medical School—a six-year-old institution with no federal funds and with no formal affiliation with any established university—became the nation's leading pregnancy research center. To underwrite the work, Hodgen sought corporate support. If the government wasn't interested, there were drug companies with products to test and a new market to capture.

In 1991, Hodgen prepared to conduct the human embryo experiments he had been forbidden to perform while still a federal scientist at NIH. He would attempt to diagnose human embryos conceived by couples who risked transmitting a hereditary disease, called Tay-Sachs, to their offspring. The lethal defect is most commonly found among Jews of East European descent. To extract a single cell for testing from each embryo, Hodgen and his Jones Institute team would use their own variation of the technique developed by Jacques Cohen to "slurp" human embryos. In lieu of federal approval, the experiment would be reviewed first by an internal medical board at the Eastern Virginia Medical School and by an outside panel of lawyers, scientists, and professional ethicists.

Even as public-health officials argued over whether laboratory conception was a fit topic of public speech for a federal scientist, doctors delivered the eighty-eighth child conceived in a laboratory dish. One hundred women were pregnant with such embryos. Thousands of couples added their names to waiting lists at the new conception clinics.

As the 1990s began, the underlying storms over reproductive control showed no signs of abating. Although the court protected the right to use birth control outside a marriage, it had yet to address directly whether there is any constitutional right to procreate by whatever technical means available. In Roe v.

Wade, a 1973 decision revolving around an unmarried woman's abortion, the Supreme Court recognized that the right to end a pregnancy, like the right to marry or raise one's own children, was a basic question of human reproductive privacy. That right, the court said, was "fundamental." Yet the justices made it contingent on technology. They linked women's reproductive privacy to medicine's ability to keep a fetus alive outside the womb. In so doing, they ceded final authority to the doctors.

Two decades after the court's landmark ruling, anti-abortion demonstrations had reached a new fever pitch, spurred in part by advances in fetal surgery and neonatal intensive-care units that improved the ability of the fetus to survive outside the womb. Doctors most closely involved in infertility treatment and reproductive research found the resurgence of the abortion debate threatening. In the years since Roe v. Wade, they transformed reproductive choice into a spectrum of possibilities. The technology of laboratory conception itself, virtually a subject for science fiction when the nine justices of the Supreme Court last directly addressed the questions posed by the beginnings of human life, had become a clinical routine. New anti-abortion laws focused the argument on conception itself, seeking to redefine the legal beginnings of life. There were already state judges willing to rule that embryos were children. A new wave of restrictive abortion statutes could extend legal protection to fertilized human eggs, sharply curtailing clinical practice and research. Galvanized by a 1989 Supreme Court decision that allowed states greater freedom to restrict abortion, membership in women's rights groups surged for the first time in years. The National Organization for Women, for example, enlisted 100,000 new members. Where two decades before, women had marched for the right to be treated no differently from men—in some instances even opposing maternity-leave policies as special treatment—they now organized more adamantly around the issue of reproductive choice and family.

Legislators of every nation were conscious that they stood at the frontier of a new creation; but they could not agree on how to conduct the journey into its uncharted territory. At least 85 national bioethical committees and law-reform commissions representing 25 countries had reviewed some or all of the reproductive technologies. More than 125 additional formal government assessments of the new reproductive techniques had been prepared, but never published. What U.S. officials handled by executive fiat, other countries confronted in an open national debate. Among the major industrialized nations, at least eight countries—home to more than 261 conception clinics—had adopted legislation to control laboratory conception. The Council of Europe drew up extensive recommendations for its member countries. The laws and commission reports revealed radically different attitudes toward human biology and the mechanics of reproducing the species. Oversight was haphazard. Regulations designed to monitor embryo research often ended up throttling it. Political interference in regulatory reviews was routine. There was no national or international consensus on research into the beginnings of human life or the appropriate application of the resulting clinical technologies.

In France, where a pregnant woman often was viewed by the central government as a kind of national hero performing a patriotic act, a national commission of scientists and philosophers urged a moratorium on advanced embryo research at the country's 100 infertility clinics because the work would encourage "ethically reprehensible attempts to standardize human reproduction for reasons of health and convenience." Laboratory conception, the ethics committee said, "accentuates the tendency to reduce human bodies to the state of instruments."

In Britain, pro-life activists and scientists clashed directly over legislation to permit embryo research and license conception clinics. "The answer is simple," said the Duke of Norfolk during the 1990 House of Lords debate. "I believe that an embryo is the start of life and must be given the same status in life as a child, a grown-up person, or a Member of your Lordships' Chamber. I can see no distinction between that and the life of an embryo." In the House of Commons, leaders formally freed party members to vote their conscience on matters concerning the sanctity of the embryo, the limits of con-

ception research, and a couple's reproductive privacy. The
bitter fight over the meaning of life resulted in a series of key
scientific and moral precedents should the U.S. Congress ever
attempt to enact comprehensive legislation on the subject. In
the end, Parliament created a single government authority to
regulate centers that store human sperm, eggs, or embryos,
and to control research on human embryos. British lawmakers
made it a criminal act to operate an IVF clinic or conduct
research without a license. They gave test-tube babies the right
to sue the doctors that created them. They authorized research
on human embryos less than 14 days old. They made it illegal
to determine the gender of an embryo for the sole purpose of
sex selection. No one would be allowed to alter the genetic
structure of an embryo. Any effort to delete harmful genes or
insert desirable ones would be illegal.

"The pro-lifers here have tried to link IVF and abortion,"
said Alan Handyside at Hammersmith Hospital. "They say I
am destroying life. They focus on the embryos we are rejecting.
We focus on the fact we are enabling a couple to have a healthy
family. We feel it is an immoral situation to permit a technique
without allowing the research that will improve it."

In April 1990, almost two years after the last deposition had
been filed, Judge Williams declared the research provision of
the Illinois law unconstitutional.

For the first time, a federal judge ruled that a woman's right
to privacy protected her privilege to seek advanced conception
technology such as in vitro fertilization, embryo micromanipulation, and genetic testing. The law had impinged "upon a
woman's right of privacy and reproductive freedom" and was
so vaguely worded that even the most well-intentioned doctor
could never be sure whether or not he was breaking the law
in question.

Embryo transfer and a prenatal testing technique called chorionic villus sampling were examples of the problem, Judge
Williams explained in her decision. "Both procedures are 'experimental' by most definitions of that term. Both are performed directly and intentionally on the fetus. Neither
procedure is necessarily therapeutic to the fetus. In embryo

transfer, it is not therapeutic to remove the embryo from a woman's uterus after it has been fertilized and expose it to the high risk associated with trying to implant it in the infertile woman. In chorionic villus sampling, it is not therapeutic to the fetus to invade and snip off some of its surrounding tissue. Both embryo transfer and chorionic villus sampling may violate any reasonable interpretation of [the law]. Both procedures, however, fall within a woman's zone of privacy . . .

"Embryo transfer is a procedure designed to enable an infertile woman to bear her own child. It takes no great leap of logic to see that within the cluster of constitutionally protected choices that include the right to have access to contraceptives, there must be included within that cluster the right to submit to a medical procedure that may bring about, rather than prevent, a pregnancy."

In the flurry of abortion cases inching toward the Supreme Court that spring, Judge Williams's ruling in Chicago drew little attention. Legal experts, however, said that her decision dramatically expanded the idea of reproductive privacy "past birthing, past pregnancy terminations, and has now reached into the sphere of reproductive technology and genetic testing." Experiments on human embryos and fetuses immediately became legal in Illinois. It made no difference to the city's infertility clinics. But within days of the decision, one Chicago hospital announced that it planned a series of transplant experiments with brain tissue from aborted fetuses. Until then, only two other centers in the United States had the will, or the private funding, to undertake such research. Whether they liked it or not, Illinois infertility specialists found themselves back in the middle of an abortion debate.

On the surface, fetal-tissue researchers had little in common with clinical practitioners of laboratory conception. One group was intent on enhancing conception to produce live babies; the other used the failures of conception to evaluate the medical potential of fetal cells. But everyone researching the beginnings of human life, in one scientist's words, "was balanced on the head of the same pin." Whether they approved of each other's work or not, infertility specialists found themselves in the same political boat with those who sought to perform research on aborted fetuses. Both were caught in the struggle over when it was permissible to end a human pregnancy.

No sooner had Judge Williams disposed of the Lifchez lawsuit than it was back in front of her again, revived by an anti-abortion activist who feared the right to experiment on embryos made every unborn child a potential victim for medical experiments.

Andrew D. Scholberg, assistant director of the Chicago-based Pro-Life Action League, sought to appeal Williams's ruling on behalf of the fetus developing in his wife's womb and all the unborn babies in Illinois, currently conceived or to be conceived in the future. Medical experiments posed a direct threat to the fetus, Scholberg's attorney argued. The judge's ruling left all such unborn children unprotected from researchers, even though the fetus "can be a patient and have rights in utero." The judge had consciously ignored the state's abortion policy and the sanctity of life of the unborn child, the attorney argued. "With the tens of thousands of abortions that have been and no doubt will be performed each year in the State of Illinois, the opinion and order place untold numbers of unborn babies at similar risk as Baby Scholberg."

Judge Williams looked down from the bench, barely disguising her disbelief. "I think it is a very bizarre reading of the court's opinion. It does not rule on the validity of the abortion law. It had nothing to do with it." Motion denied. A minute ticked by.

The lawyers headed for the hall. They would be back—if not in this courtroom or for this case, then another. The judge considered her ruling definitive, but for attorneys on both sides of the abortion issue it was just one more legal skirmish in a larger battle.

Those most concerned about the sanctity of human life had only succeeded in placing lives at risk.

What the public research moratorium cost could not be measured in dollars or derailed careers. It left thousands of men and women who conceived families through the new technology with no independent authority to protect their health or the health of their children. The federal watchdogs who protected an earlier generation of American children from the ravages of thalidomide were effectively muzzled.

"You don't have any federal involvement because there is no research. You don't have any oversight from insurance companies because most companies won't cover it at all. The absence of these things has left it all in an arena where no one is watching," said congressional investigator D. Ann Murphy.

With virtually no federal public-health support, by 1990 U.S. researchers had completed only one limited study to determine the long-term health of the children produced through laboratory conception. Doctors who studied 83 children conceived at the Jones Institute through in vitro fertilization found that test-tube babies were just as healthy and alert as infants conceived naturally. The children were all between twelve and thirty months old at the time of the 1989 study. In England, researchers reviewed more than 1,000 test-tube births at Bourn Hall and found no significant developmental defects. Any birth defects, like the high numbers of abnormal IVF embryos, were blamed on maternal age or the physical condition that caused the couples' initial infertility. These were, after all, high-risk pregnancies, the researchers reminded their colleagues. It was unclear what such studies, surveying the children produced by the world's two most experienced clinics, revealed about a field in which procedures and success rates varied widely among clinics.

While such limited studies settled any immediate fears about the health of test-tube babies, they did little to quiet misgivings about long-term health consequences of the fertility drugs and laboratory techniques required to conceive a child outside the body. They did nothing to assess the health effects on the women who went through the procedures. Some subtle side effects might take decades to develop. The physical defects and cancers caused by DES, for example, appeared only after the children or grandchildren reached puberty. So much time elapsed before the first DES symptoms appeared that it was often impossible to establish a direct link to the drug. Prescription slips had been thrown away. Medical records were lost. The mothers who took DES and the doctors who prescribed it often had died of old age. Without meticulous records, it was almost impossible to link cause and effect. Researchers faced the same problem when they uncovered evidence that linked prenatal amniocentesis to a higher incidence of childhood ear infections. Scientists surmised that the withdrawal of amniotic fluid for testing might cause pressure changes in the ear that "perturbed anatomical development." But, without detailed medical records, they couldn't be certain about the connection.

Scientists trying to assess the long-term effects of fertility drugs found themselves in the same quandary. More than 20 years after it was approved for marketing, researchers were raising questions about the safety of the most commonly used fertility drug in the United States. Biologists from the University of California at San Francisco found evidence that clomiphene citrate, the artificial hormone that under the Dow trade name "Clomid" and the Serono trade name "Serophene" had been prescribed to millions of women since the 1960s, could interfere with the normal development of a fetus in the womb. The studies were conducted with human fetal tissue and laboratory mice. The scientists weren't sure how to determine the margin of safety for women who may take the fertility drug for years or in the course of multiple cycles of in vitro fertilization.

"I have become very concerned that the fertility drugs of the 1980s and the 1990s will become the next DES story," said Lucinda Finley at the State University of New York. "DES was supposedly going to help reduce miscarriages and make babies bigger and healthier. In the postwar baby boom, it was greeted by everyone as this great wonder drug that was only going to help society. Nobody knows how many women are DES-exposed because there aren't good records. Now, partly because of DES, we have a generation of women who are having trouble getting pregnant. Now it is the drugs that help people get pregnant that are being greeted with such enthusiasm. Women are being pumped up with these, without really knowing the long-term effects. I get very sobered by how little the pharmaceutical industry learns from each of its disasters."

Clomiphene is a synthetic estrogen compound given to infertile women to stimulate release of a pituitary hormone that in turn triggers the ovary to release an egg. The drug is usually prescribed for women who don't ovulate or who don't have normal hormonal output after ovulating. Many physicians, however, prescribe the drug for infertile women in general, or if they cannot diagnose the cause of infertility. Women usually stop taking clomiphene before they become pregnant, but evidence suggested that the drug could remain in the body for weeks afterward. If levels remain high enough during the time the fetal reproductive tract is developing, it may—like DES—cross the placenta to the fetus, where it could have harmful effects, including malformations of the vagina, uterus, and fallopian tubes. Officials at Merrell Dow Pharmaceuticals, which makes clomiphene, said they have monitored the drug for two decades and found no evidence of birth defects. Properly prescribed and properly administered, the drug should offer no cause for concern. They said, however, that it may be too soon to detect long-term adverse effects because the children of the women who took the drug are only now reaching their childbearing years. Similar questions hang over other drugs administered to enhance a woman's fertility or arrest diseases of the reproductive tract.

Clomiphene typically is given for only five days of a woman's ovulatory cycle, beginning four days after the onset of menstruation. Since ovulation occurs about 14 or 15 days into the cycle, most women stop taking the drug a week before fertilization occurs. Some physicians, however, recommend taking large doses of clomiphene up to 25 days into the cycle. Drug company studies indicate that 40 days after the last dose of clomiphene was administered, the amount of the drug still in the bloodstream was quite low. Researchers, however, suspect that such measurements may be misleading because they indicate only how much of the drug is in the blood, not in the body's tissues or in the uterus itself, where, like the estrogen it chemically mimics, clomiphene would be expected to concentrate. Consequently, when the fetal reproductive tract begins to develop in the sixth week of gestation, concentrations of the drug in the uterus might be dangerously high, even though total body levels of the drug may be well within safety limits.

"I look at my little babies and I think: Well, they are healthy now, but what about in twenty years? I worry about them. Actually, I am more worried about my health," said a cancer specialist who is the mother of test-tube twins.

While undergoing her third in vitro fertilization attempt in 1989, she watched two former infertility patients be diagnosed with breast cancer at the hospital where she worked.

"They had gone through repeated rounds of Clomid and Pergonal in order to conceive. They found their breast lumps while they were breast-feeding their babies. I watched one of these women die, leaving behind her fourteen-month-old baby. I can't think of anything worse than to go through all this to have a baby and then die while it was young." As she watched her own babies learn to crawl, she worried about the effects of the fertility drugs she had taken. "I don't even talk to my husband about this—about what this may have done to my health in the long run. Breast cancer is already epidemic among women my age. I don't think we know the carcinogenic effects of those drugs as well as we should or as well as we will when people like me are fifty years old. I probably have a higher risk of breast cancer. I think we may find that a lot of women who go through this will have a higher risk of breast cancer, leukemia, lymphomas, or other cancers of the repro-ductive system. You can't tell me that there aren't things about the impact of those drugs on newly developing cells in your body that we don't fully understand yet. I have to wonder about the effects of repeated IVF cycles, about repeated ex-posures to high levels of these drugs like Clomid, Pergonal, Metrodin, Progesterone, Danazol, and God knows what else I've taken. How many other people like me are out there whose medical histories aren't being followed?"

There was no reported link between fertility drugs and breast or other cancers, only the fear of the women who took them for months or years at a time. Pharmaceutical companies that did maintain comprehensive patient records were under no obligation to share all their information. Not until 1988 did the federal government take the first step to assess the long-term safety of laboratory conception, when the National Institute for Child Health and Development signed a five-year contract to collect health information on 13,000 women undergoing laboratory conception procedures at nine U.S. infertility clinics. It might be a decade or more before the results were known. The registry would only track the long-term health of women, not the children they conceived. Even in Australia, where a national birth register noted every child born as a result of laboratory conception, no one knew what happened after mother and child left the hospital. There was no money for systematic follow-up.

"Women who enter the program should be sent a question-naire five, ten, and twenty-five years after their treatment," said Dr. Barbara Burton, president of the Infertility Federation of Australia. "No one has long-term statistics on IVF children, either.

"When you are involved in infertility groups," she said, "you hear things casually on the grapevine. For instance, one baby developed a tumor when he was one year old. That sort of thing tends to make you worry. Does it have anything to do with IVF? If there was follow-up, we might find out there was no need to worry."

Would subtle developmental defects turn up among IVF children? No one knew. No one seemed anxious to ask. Each newborn, when it came into the world, was such a gift to its parents that to question its origins seemed more than the heart could bear.

The life and death of Christopher Duda was such a story. He and his sister, Danielle, born seconds apart at Evanston Hospital outside Chicago on May 14, 1983, were the nation's second test-tube twins. They were the product of their parents' third try at in vitro fertilization. The newborn girl was perfectly healthy, but her brother was born without a spleen and with only two chambers in his heart, instead of four. His defective heart hindered the flow of blood to his lungs; the lack of a spleen undermined his defenses against infection. He under-went his first of four major heart operations when he was two days old. He died when he was seven. Doctors said they had no way of knowing whether the birth defects were related to in vitro fertilization. "We can speculate that it might have been a contributing factor, but there is no evidence," an attending cardiac surgeon told reporters.

The father, Robert Duda, consoled himself with the thought that after he and his wife had been told they would never have any children, technology had blessed them with two.

"The miracle is that I had a beautiful son for seven years," he said.

11

Mine to Hold

The clinical trial was almost over.

Neither the doctors nor the couples who volunteered for Jacques Cohen's embryo experiment could see yet how their part in it would end. After a half-dozen failures, some couples wondered whether the laboratory was any better than their own barren bodies. When it came, a positive pregnancy test was a reprieve.

For Pam Roberts, the telephone rang at her office nine days before her thirty-fifth birthday. "I started screaming before the nurse could say anything. I got out of my chair and started jumping up and down. Over the telephone, I could hear all the nurses at the clinic clapping. I was so excited I couldn't think of my husband's telephone number. As soon as he picked up the phone, I started screaming. I didn't even say anything. After all that hell, finally, finally it had paid off. Within an hour and a half, the florist delivered a dozen red roses from my husband. He had never sent me flowers before."

Lisa Boone, thirty-one, convinced herself she was pregnant even before she went in for the test. The numbers confirmed what her body had already told her.

"I was just so high thinking that it had worked, but I was very hush-hush. I didn't let anybody know what I was thinking or what I was feeling because I didn't want to disappoint my husband or my parents or anybody else. The clinic called me and said, 'We have great news for you. You have a positive pregnancy test.' I just wanted to tell everybody that I was pregnant, but I didn't, not until I was well beyond the danger zone. So I was trying to hide it. I didn't wear maternity clothes. I actually waited almost four months to tell anybody that I was pregnant."

In the first weeks, their pregnancies were cryptic readouts on a sensitive chemical assay. Some clinics swelled their success statistics with such biochemical pregnancies, but only about three-quarters of them normally resulted in the birth of a child. The Boones and the Robertses shared their lives with a developing fetus whose most tangible presence in its first weeks was a string of numbers read over the telephone. The other couples lived with disappointment.

Susan and David Parr, the weekend sailors, had four frozen embryos in storage. She still couldn't face another cycle of laboratory conception. "I'm fried from all this," she said. The more she distanced herself from the process, the better she felt. The fertility drugs slowly leached from her system. She dieted away the pounds she had gained while undergoing in vitro fertilization. For the first time in years, she liked what she saw in the mirror. Her husband no longer seemed like an enemy. "We are nearing the end," he said. "We have gone through everything. We will have gallantly tried. We don't want to become one of those people who—kicking, screaming, and begging—ask the doctor to do it again."

Dana and John Hobart booked themselves on another cruise. Maybe their failure to conceive would seem less important from a sundeck overlooking the Caribbean. If they found the money and the stamina to try another cycle of in vitro fertilization, they would have to start from scratch. They had exhausted their store of frozen embryos; they had exhausted themselves. On the other hand, they were hopeful about adoption. Their attorney had located an unmarried college student who was six months pregnant. She might be willing to offer her child for adoption. The lawyer gave her the files of five couples to read and from which to choose a set of parents. The Hobarts's chances were almost exactly the same as in laboratory conception—one in five.

Lisa and Bill Fagg, the Resolve volunteers, could tell them that adoption was no easier. Couples had to tread carefully through a thicket of adoption regulations or they could find themselves in jail. One Florida woman was arrested and charged with a felony after she paid $3,000 for another woman's newborn daughter in what was essentially a private adoption transaction. Bill and Lisa paid close attention to their lawyer's advice. In April, only a few weeks before the birth of the baby they expected to adopt, the birth mother vanished. "She had an appointment for an ultrasound and didn't show up," Lisa Fagg explained. "She went to see her family and never came back. She had apparently never told her mother she was pregnant. When she did, her mother talked her into keeping the baby."

They were left holding a cradle. They would have to find some other way to fill it. The months had moved them higher on the waiting list at the Catholic Social Services adoption agency. They had five frozen embryos in storage. To their friends, they bore their disappointment lightly. But when she had to sit through a baby shower several days later, Lisa felt her smile freeze in place like a fright mask.

In the days that followed her pregnancy test, Pam Roberts watched her hormone levels soar. *Jesus! How many babies are in there?* she wondered. Within a few weeks, she would know. The technicians could trace the sonic shadow of the developing infant with the same kind of ultrasound probe they had used to find her ripe eggs. They could monitor the minute flutter of the heart.

"When we went for our first ultrasound, we saw the first little baby and the first little heartbeat," Pam said. "The technician said: 'There it is.' Larry told her to keep looking. There were two." When Lisa Boone went for her first ultrasound test, she also saw two hearts flicker on the video monitor. Her own heart skipped a beat.

To their collection of embryo photographs, the expectant couples added a print of the sonogram picture. The black-and-silver ultrasound image was as inscrutable as the face in the Shroud of Turin—a blurred picture of an answered prayer.

Lisa Boone and Pam Roberts were themselves almost twins. Both were blond, extroverted, energetic. Each was a driven executive responsible for scores of employees. Lisa Boone managed the Vinings Club, an exclusive private restaurant and health club on the outskirts of Atlanta. Pam Roberts managed the outpatient oncology department at Northside Hospital a few blocks from the clinic. Each had married a lawyer. David Boone, thirty-five, specialized in malpractice claims. Larry Roberts, thirty-nine, was a patent attorney who specialized in medical technology. Before they wed, both couples had known they could not conceive unaided. In three years of marriage, the Boones went through IVF twice. In their four years together, the Roberts had tried five times. Both couples had volunteered to have their eggs and embryos surgically altered. Each woman was convinced that Cohen's "hatching" microsurgery had given her the extra edge that finally made her pregnant.

But it was a blind trial. One couple's embryos were an unaltered control group; the other had undergone the experimental micromanipulation. Neither woman really knew for certain which she nurtured within her womb. Neither did their doctors.

Lisa Boone hoped her pregnancy would help recapture the intimacy and romance that infertility treatments had stripped from her marriage. What they had lost as husband and wife, she hoped they would find as a mother and father. "I thought that everything would be almost a fairy tale—that we would go through this process, however clinical it was, to get pregnant and then, once we were pregnant, we would cross the line to become normal people. We would be happy together and pick out things for the baby's crib together and talk about names, talk about diapers, and all the things that I thought expectant parents would think about and talk about. I wanted everything to be so normal. So textbook," she said. "Actually, it almost wrecked my marriage."

Later, David Boone would remember his anger and isolation. Lisa Boone would remember her anguish and her own loneliness. "You don't want to trade your wife for kids," he would say. "But when you get the idea of kids, you almost would not trade anything for your ability to have them." When she became pregnant, she thought technology had solved their problems. It was only then, however, that they could recognize how deeply technology had driven the wedge between them.

She was a general's daughter—tall, athletic, with long, streaked blond hair and a low, husky voice. He was a litigator who loved to fly. His high forehead, wavy brown hair, and freckles set off his shrewd and sleepy blue eyes. David and Lisa Boone were the perfect power couple, always on their way to his Cessna for a quick flight to the next concert, a beach house, or a favorite ski slope. When they could not agree on a restaurant during one of their first dates, he flew her on the spur of the moment to Asheville, North Carolina, where they ate barbecue at the airport diner.

They loved their work almost as much as each other. Twelve-hour days; six-day weeks. They reveled in each new career coup—his next million-dollar malpractice verdict; her next successful marketing strategy. "Everything has always worked for me in life, one way or another," he said. His family called him "Perfect David." Her father called her "Super-Chick."

He planned her seduction with the care of a seasoned Casanova and all the nervous anticipation of a giddy teenager. The maid cleaned his house twice. He filled the rooms with candlelight and set the table for a six-course dinner: veal Marsala, three kinds of wine. They were in each other's arms before dessert. "Do you just want to live with me forever or do you want to marry me?" she asked him one evening. He was skittish, since he'd been married and divorced twice before. She had never been married. When he proposed, he gave her a diamond-studded ring with the family crest.

A pelvic infection in her junior year of college, misdiagnosed by a campus clinician, left Lisa unable to conceive unaided.

At least 10 percent of the women who contract pelvic inflammatory disease are left infertile after a single episode. He wanted whatever family they could have, and he was willing to adopt. Even though she knew her chances were remote, she wanted to conceive their own baby.

"I knew that if I wanted to have kids, it was going to have to be through extraordinary measures," she said. "I wanted to have a child because it would be our child, because we were very much in love. Just having a kid was not my objective—we didn't need that to be complete. So adopting one just to have a kid was not what I wanted to do." Whatever hard work and money could accomplish, they were willing to try. Conception was another challenge, another hurdle to clear.

After their honeymoon, she underwent laser surgery. Tests and more tests. More pelvic surgery. Laparoscopy. Laparotomy. David followed along in the medical textbooks. In 1989, they decided to try in vitro fertilization. They volunteered to have her eggs surgically altered. They agreed to have their embryos "hatched." They consented to have their excess embryos frozen.

"We felt that whatever these doctors thought was the right thing to be doing with our eggs was fine, because the whole process of in vitro in itself was, for the most part, experimental," she said. "Naturally, I had all the concerns that probably any woman does: Will my baby be deformed? Is this going to screw up the chromosomal balance? You're playing with a real special balance of ingredients and you don't want to think they're doing something that's Frankensteinish."

For her first egg retrieval, they arrived at the clinic at 11 A.M. on the dot. They were ready; the clinic was not. The procedure had been postponed until 12:30. The doctor was another hour late. All but two of the resulting embryos were abnormal. David and Lisa were convinced the two-hour delay was the cause. The two normal embryos were placed inside her, but they did not survive.

The distraught couple kept waiting to hear from the doctor: an apology, regrets, anything. "We never saw him again after the day he was two hours late for the retrieval," she said. What they did see were his bills. They signed checks for thousands week after week. Then, almost 16 months after the procedure had been performed and the last bill paid, one $48 invoice appeared in the mail. It was the doctor's last word. They were enraged.

The bitterness from their first failure rose like a wall between them. David sent her flowers. "You could set her up for something she can't ever produce, and then she could feel that great disappointment. You risked making her think that if she didn't have a child she was less than one hundred percent of what you wanted life to be with her. On the other hand, if you completely pull away and didn't give any support to the project, then it looked like you didn't care if you did have a baby. So you tried to find some middle ground.

"I tried to make her feel it didn't matter to me," David said. "The failure of the in vitro attempt did not take a baby away from me. It took away my wife. There was nothing more important to me. I am a high-maintenance partner. I wanted my wife back." He convinced himself that he didn't matter enough to her. "She busied herself with non-baby things and non-family things and non-David things. Men need respect and adoration, and I wasn't being adored. I was being put out with the cat. The adoration was put on hold while she protected herself from what she had been through, like cells in a body surrounding a splinter," he said. "I was angry and I swallowed it."

When they came home from work, they avoided each other. They ate in silence and fell asleep watching television.

"Here is a 'super-chick' who can't have kids. They did the magic and it didn't work. I buried myself in work. She buried herself."

More and more often, he was away on business. She arranged for her friends to administer her daily hormone injections. "I was just like: Fine. Go. Be away. I'd just as soon do this myself," she said. She took a ski vacation and didn't invite him. They no longer made love. When she signed up again for in vitro fertilization, the decision was hers. They hadn't discussed the idea.

"I was not consulted," he said. "I was advised after the decision had been made. I was not a part of it. She had shut me out of the process. That was a very large blow to me." He burrowed deeper into work. He tried seven lawsuits in eight weeks. He was married to his schedule: court dates, depositions, strategy meetings. She was married to hers: hormone shots, ultrasound scans, urine tests.

When she went through her second egg retrieval, he was in court in Florida. The doctors at Reproductive Biology Associates retrieved eight eggs. "Then I was told, at a certain day and a certain time, I was supposed to come in a jar. Boy, I certainly felt special then," David said. "I think that is as close as you can get to feeling what women say they feel when a guy has disappeared after a one-night stand. I think they even asked if I could Federal Express my stuff from Florida."

Six eggs fertilized; two others were polyspermic. Jacques Cohen surgically altered four of the embryos and froze two others. David was in town only long enough to watch the embryo transfer, and then was gone again. Two weeks later, when the clinic called with the results of the pregnancy test, Lisa Boone had her husband on hold on the other line. He was in West Palm Beach trying a case.

She relayed the news. "Guess what! The rabbit died!" she told him.

"Good for you," he replied.

"What do you mean, 'Good for me'? Good for us," she said.

There was silence at the other end of the phone. The distance between them was no longer simply physical; a rift had grown that a baby alone could not bridge.

"I thought I had just been sentenced to life imprisonment," David recalled. "The feeling I always had about wanting children was nowhere that I could grab onto and take solace in. I felt like I had just been told, 'Your wife and your child are going to run the rest of your life and you are not going to be in charge of anything.' I was drifting away. Nothing she did was going to get me back."

She went to the first ultrasound by herself. When the sonogram revealed two heartbeats, David was elated about the pregnancy for the first time.

"There was a tweak of excitement," he said. But it still seemed the work of a stranger. He was just semen in a plastic cup, he would joke to his friends; a whack-off dad. Every time Lisa heard the punch line she winced. Six weeks after the first sonogram, the ultrasound scan revealed that one of the developing twins was gone. Two heartbeats had become one.

"I hate to even admit this, but I even considered aborting the child," she said later. "Things were that bad between us. I had gotten pregnant because I had wanted to be a parent with him. For a short period of time, I thought—regardless of how much I had been through to get pregnant—that I didn't want a child if it wasn't with him."

To support the pregnancy, she still took daily injections of Progesterone. Emotional support came from her obstetrician and the nurses at RBA.

"I had a husband who was about ready not to be my husband anymore. I was just a mess. I remember thinking: How could he do this to me after what we've been through?" Their heartache fed on itself. Then she realized that she had helped to push him away. The commitment they had made to their marriage and to each other, stretched by the strain, held strong. With luck and love, they found each other. Friends helped, as did an astute psychologist.

"I don't believe I was mad at Lisa," he said. "I don't believe I was mad at the fact that Lisa had an infection. I don't think I was mad at any of that stuff. I think my male ego had been harmed because of the dreams I had grown up with. You think you are going to look at someone, fall passionately in love with that someone, set up house, make wild love and produce, from the product of that love, a baby. The biggest thing that you can do if you love someone else is have their children. Part of the anger I went through was not being able to make my baby that way."

In its final months, their pregnancy was redemptive. "It was a different life. I was very happy she was in me," said Lisa Boone. "When she would kick me or when I could talk with somebody else about being pregnant, I really loved it. David was making time for her and for me. We did more things together. He traveled less. We went to childbirth classes. We began to do things much more together." She had no physical complications to contend with, but she worried about losing their child. "I didn't want to run or exercise. I didn't want to jump up and down because I was afraid it was going to fall out. I was very tentative. I remember we were up in Maine for Labor Day weekend. My best girlfriend and her husband were there. She was pregnant and I just still felt like mine wasn't normal yet. I was jealous. She could take long, hard walks. They could have intercourse.

"They had conceived naturally. I still felt like ours was supernatural," she said.

Pam and Larry Roberts settled in to enjoy the months of what her new obstetrician called this "premium" pregnancy that had cost $30,000 to achieve. There had never been a moment in their married life unaffected by the struggle to conceive. Now they could throw away the ovulation kits and halt the hormone injections. The moment had come to choose nursery colors; watch breasts and belly swell; try on maternity clothes; buy strollers; arrange maternity leave.

"I had been ready to give up," she said. "It was our fifth attempt. It took every bit of gut and emotion we had. Wonderful things can come from terrible pain." And now, she thought, the pain was over. Pregnancy would heal them.

With such thoughts, Pam Roberts lulled herself to sleep each night. One morning in her ninth week of pregnancy, she awoke before dawn to prepare for an early morning business meeting. In the bathroom, she found herself soaked with blood.

"I thought I had been frightened before, but I had never known such fear. My hands were sweating. My heart was racing. I couldn't think." She could not staunch the hemorrhage. Had she miscarried? Larry drove her to the doctor's office. "All I knew was that when I got there I wanted to see two heartbeats," she said. The hearts winked on the screen—Baby A, Baby B. The bleeding continued on and off for three weeks.

"We were relieved, but now we were scared shitless," she said. "We thought getting pregnant was the battle, and we had won it. We didn't realize that was only the first half of the battle. I remember both of us being so nervous and depressed because we thought: This is only the beginning. Now we have nine more months of pure fear."

A generation ago, most women had given birth to their last child before women like Lisa Boone or Pam Roberts conceived their first. Improved medical care made delayed childbirth safer than ever. Although healthy older women are no more likely to encounter complications than younger women, there are extra risks. Older women having their first baby face an increased risk of toxemia, a blood condition that can threaten the life of the mother and the baby. Babies born to mothers with toxemia have five times the risk of dying before birth or as newborns. Older women also are more likely to develop placental problems that could result in smaller or premature babies. As women age, they face an increased risk of developing high blood pressure, diabetes, or some other health problem that might complicate a pregnancy. With proper medical care, the conditions could be managed. And there was no evidence that working throughout pregnancy put a baby in any danger.

Multiple embryos, however, put themselves at risk. Common enough among women in their late thirties, twins had become epidemic among couples who conceived with the aid of fertility drugs or through in vitro fertilization. In 1989, more twins were born in the United States than ever before. One well-to-do Atlanta neighborhood was typical. Within a few blocks of one another, there were three sets of IVF twins and one set of IVF triplets.

About half of all twins would be born premature. Even those that were carried to full term were more likely to be born underweight and often faced weeks of hospital care. The women who bore them were more likely to become anemic, to have high blood pressure, or to hemorrhage. The delivery itself could be so complicated that half of all twins were delivered by caesarean section.

"My OB outlined how they managed a woman who was thirty-five with a twin pregnancy . . . how they wanted you to eat, the fact that you were not to exercise at all," Pam Roberts said. "You could walk moderately, but no aerobic walking, no power walking, no jogging, no sit-ups, no anything because of the threat of miscarriage and abortion. They would monitor you intensively with ultrasound and lab tests. At twenty-six weeks I would go on bed rest. A multiple-pregnancy IVF mom at thirty-five was high risk to them. I reduced my workload and cut out travel. I canceled speeches. They didn't want me to sit for prolonged periods, so we didn't even go to the movies. We were scared to death."

Nonetheless, Larry Roberts was relieved to become a father. "People talk about the biological clock ticking as if it were a female phenomena. I feel I went through that," he said. His blue eyes glinted behind a pair of wire-rim aviator glasses. He was cordial, reserved, a big man who carried his bulk discreetly. "I didn't want to be on Social Security when my children were in Little League. I would wake up in a cold sweat wondering what I was going to do about it. She knew I wanted children, biological children. She knew I did not want to adopt." He laughed. "I suppose it's one of the ultimate forms of narcissism." For both of them, it was a second marriage.

They had met once in 1978 in Augusta, Georgia, but never exchanged more than a nod. Years passed before they really spoke. She was new in Atlanta, and he was newly divorced. Mutual friends urged her to call him, but she was wary. "I wasn't going to rehabilitate any more emotionally crippled men," she recalled. "I was really sick of all that. I thought: Well, I should give him a call because it's hard to go through a divorce. I knew, because I had gone through that." She left a message on his answering machine.

They met for a drink at Friday's. They were deliberately low-key; cautious. He invited her to dinner at his apartment later that week. When she arrived, she found him standing in a flooded kitchen with his trousers rolled up; the water pipes had burst. They waded to the dining room and sat down to eat. At that moment the building maintenance crew arrived to vacuum up the water. "It sounded like 747's were in the kitchen while we were trying to eat. I guess I knew then our life wouldn't be easy," he said. It was January 1985.

She had been diagnosed with endometriosis right before they started dating. The disease, which affects four to six million American women, causes painful cramps, bleeding, and infertility. If the disease continued unchecked, she faced the likelihood that she eventually might have to undergo a hysterectomy, in which her uterus and both ovaries would be removed. A year later, she made her first appointment with Hilton Kort. He offered her a choice: laser surgery to remove the benign web of tissue and adhesions the disease had woven around her internal organs, or extended treatment with a powerful derivative of a male sex hormone called Danazol to shrink the diseased tissue. The drug, a steroid extracted from testosterone, would stop her menstrual cycle and cause a false menopause. If she elected surgery, she could expect to lose six weeks of work at a time when she could least afford it. If she chose the drug, she risked side effects that included weight gain, muscle pain, and masculinization. Some researchers suspected that it also affected the immune system.

She didn't know which was worse. Before she could make up her mind, she needed to know whether she had any future with Larry. "If we're seriously considering getting married, I need to do something now because I'm losing my fertility every month. The scar tissue is getting worse," she told him. "If we are not, I will keep taking pain pills until I can find time for the surgery." There was no graceful way to test the waters; she plunged in over her head. Yes, he was serious. Yes, he wanted children. No, he would not adopt. "I felt that if I wanted this man in my life I needed to do something to preserve my fertility," she said. That meant something sooner rather than later. She asked him to have his semen analyzed. She had the first of what would be eight months' worth of Danazol prescriptions filled. "We were both still single. This was killing our relationship," she recalled. To help them handle the medical stress, they saw a counselor.

They seemed to do things backward. They found themselves in treatment for infertility before they were even engaged. They sought marriage counseling before they were married. They built a house together and then had a wedding.

The drug was worse than she expected. It transformed her body. "I had horrible, horrible mood swings. Hot flashes. An eighteen- to twenty-pound weight gain. Broke out in rashes. Was nauseated for the entire eight months I took it. I'd be up in the middle of the night vomiting. It decreased breast size. I'm a fairly well endowed lady and I was flat as a pancake. I had muscles in my legs that looked like a football player's."

They were engaged in August 1986 and married three months later. They moved into their new house three weeks before the wedding. She took the last of her Danazol two days before the ceremony. A laparoscopy after the honeymoon revealed the drug had done nothing to alleviate the disease.

"At that point, Kort recommended that we begin immediately to try to conceive. And as I remember, Larry and I looked at each other. He's thinking: We need time to be married. I'm thinking: Larry, we don't have time.

"Within two months of the wedding, we have ovulation-predictor kits all over the house. Our kitchen looked like a science lab. I'm taking Clomid, which is giving me hot flashes and making me moody. We went right from one hormone to another. We are having intercourse on a schedule which is driving both of us nuts. We are both very loving, sexual people and this took every bit of the intimacy, romance, and spontaneity out of our sexual behavior. I remember watching the 'Today' show with my feet up on Larry's back after intercourse. I kept telling myself it was worth it because he didn't want to adopt a baby. But I didn't get pregnant."

Medical innovations were the raw material of his patent practice. By the time he and his wife conceived their twins, Larry Roberts felt as if his marriage was a well-worn proving ground. "We've tried it all," he said. "We tried IVF. We tried GIFT. We tried frozen. We tried fresh. I feel I have been paying for their experimental work. This technology is very much evolving. If they had all the answers, they wouldn't be changing it all the time. One of the things that was always a source of concern to me was that I had understood it was tried and proven technology, not something that was still highly experimental. With high hopes and desperation, maybe you hear what you want to hear."

Jacques Cohen made it clear to them that at least the "hatching" microsurgery was highly experimental. When Pam Roberts became pregnant, they were convinced that hatching was the reason why. But they wondered whether the experiment, their age, or the luck of the genetic lottery would cause a birth defect in the developing twins. Neither Larry nor Pam knew whether they could abort the twins they had struggled so hard to create. They would not be certain until amniocentesis had been performed to assess their health. Only then were the parents willing to believe in the children they created.

"Both of us made a conscious decision not to decorate a nursery," she said. "I would not even go look at anything having to do with a nursery until after the amnio. I think I had bought only two maternity dresses for work. I thought: I am not going to buy a room full of baby furniture or a bunch of clothes and have to take them back. Genetic counseling in itself was frightening, to hear about the fact that once you are thirty-five we had a one-in-three hundred chance of Down's syndrome in one of the two babies, and all the multitude of other diseases. They discuss all the things amniocentesis will tell you, and then they let you know a multitude of things that amnio won't show you.

"We talked a lot about what we would do. I am very pro-choice, but I don't know how I could have gone through an abortion. I don't know if Larry could have, either. I will fight to the death for women to have the right to have an abortion, but after all the investment we had made, I don't know what I would have done. If it had been a Down's baby, it would have been a very hard decision to make.

"Once we got the green light from the amnio, I went nuts. Then I really felt like we could celebrate. That's when we started to talk more about 'he' and 'she,' about the little boy and the little girl. We started talking about names. They took on a meaning in our lives that was separate and apart from something you wish for but never really hope to have."

After four attempts at in vitro fertilization in 13 months and $28,000 in medical bills, Lisa and Bill Fagg became parents with a telephone call. An unmarried college senior picked them to raise her newborn child.

They discovered they had become a mother and father so abruptly that when the adoption agency notified them, Lisa initially could not make sense of the conversation. "Tell me about your cradle," the caseworker said on the telephone. "Will it hold an eight-pound baby boy?"

The adoption worker was studiously nonchalant. Lisa started screaming.

The call came on a Wednesday. They saw the baby for the first time on Thursday. "When you meet him, you do have the option of saying no. We took one look at him and knew he was our son. He was the baby we waited so long to have," Lisa said. On Friday they took him home. Friends had covered the lawn in front of their apartment building with balloons. She carried the baby to the front door. They called out to her: Hey, Mom! She caught her breath. "Oh, I really am, aren't I?" she said. "I'm finally not Aunt Lisa anymore."

In the four years they had been on the agency's waiting list, the adoption fee had increased from $9,000 to $14,000. Court papers and filing fees cost $200. For a couple who placed their name on the agency's list now, the average wait was said to be seven years.

Many couples hoped to adopt their child as soon after birth as possible. The Alan Guttmacher Institute estimated that there were 1.5 million unwanted babies born in the United States every year. Only two percent of them were placed for adoption. The Child Welfare League of America counted more than 25,000 children on official adoption lists. Half of them were minorities, many were already entering elementary school, and almost all of them had "special needs." For every healthy, white baby offered for adoption, there were, by one estimate, 40 childless couples waiting in line.

In Georgia, the League counted 443 children on official adoption waiting lists; yet in an average year, more than 2,500 adoptions took place in the state. Prospective parents and private adoption attorneys scoured the country for available infants. Many had their best luck abroad. According to the Immigration and Naturalization Service, more than 9,200 foreign-born children were adopted every year, 75 percent of them from Asian countries. Not every successful adoption had a happy ending. Every year, at least 1,000 children were returned to the adoption agencies that placed them.

Before Catholic Social Services would approve them as adoptive parents, Bill and Lisa filled out more than 50 pages of forms: marriage license, birth certificates, biographies, financial statements, family histories, photographs for the birth mother. "They also want to know about your expectations, what you thought being a parent would be like," she said. "Suddenly you weren't focused on having a baby. You were focused on raising one."

The child who would be baptized Joshua William Fagg was born by caesarean section on April 23, 1990. He weighed seven pounds, three ounces. His birth mother had shiny dark hair, large hazel eyes, and a sprinkle of freckles across the bridge of her nose. His birth father had green eyes and his brown hair was thick and curly. She was, like Lisa, Catholic. He was, like Bill, Presbyterian.

"My eyes look just like his daddy's," Lisa said.

She learned his eye color from the biography he placed on record with the adoption agency. The two couples never met.

With the baby came a thick file on his birth parents—medical and genetic histories that covered the families for several generations. Whatever Bill and Lisa knew about his birth parents, they would tell their son when he was old enough: that she was shy, had skin that sunburned easily, and had a weakness for cherry pies; that he wanted to join the armed services, that his olive skin made him glow from the sun even in gray winter.

"Those are not the kind of secrets you need to keep," Lisa Fagg said. "I think you have to be very open with adoption. From a very young age, you have to let them know they are adopted. He will know exactly why they did what they did. To me, she is a pretty wonderful person because she gave us our son."

The birth mother left two presents for the child she would never see again—a crucifix and a yellow, hand-woven baby blanket.

"She had one just like it when she was born. It was her way of closing the door. It was like a ceremony to wrap it to give to us; everything had to be perfect. It really moved me," Lisa said. The birth mother's parents had enclosed a baptismal prayer that hung now with the crucifix over the baby's crib. They left him letters to mark the place he held in their hearts.

In black ink on onionskin paper, the grandparents wrote: "He is our first grandson and now we may never see him again. We did have a few days in the hospital, after the birth, to share him with our daughter. We proceeded hesitantly at first, but soon felt very comfortable with him—each of us taking turns holding him, rocking him, feeding, changing diapers, loving. We knew we would have to crowd years of emotions into those few precious days." They added: "We ask for your prayers for our daughter—she has begun the grief process and will need time for healing."

On plain white foolscap, the daughter typed: "I feel happiness and joy for our son and his new parents, and sadness for my loss. I find great comfort every time I think of our son and the life he will lead with both of you as his parents. I thank the Lord for our son's life and for allowing me to bring him into this world. I cherish the five days I was able to spend with our son in the hospital. . . . I pray that someday our son will want to contact me. I understand that this must be his choice. Our son will always be my firstborn child and will always be in my heart and in my thoughts and in my prayers. . . . I wish your family happiness and love always."

Bill and Lisa kept the letters in a plain manila folder along with the adoption papers. "He's going to come home someday and say: Did I come from your belly, Mommy? That file is his answer. That is his information. That file belongs to him, not us," he said.

They watched the baby learn to roll his way across the floor.

"He's our son," Bill said. "He is our life."

Lisa wrote a letter to his birth mother. Bill was working on a letter to the birth mother's parents, who were about his age. That would end their contact.

They knew they still had other family obligations. There were five frozen embryos at Reproductive Biology Associates; they had been in storage for a year now. The clinic periodically mailed them reminders. "They are future possiblities of children for us," she said. "I don't want to keep them in limbo. We aren't getting any younger. I want to see if there are any changes in technology that can help us come up with brothers or sisters for Joshua.

"Emotionally and physically, I don't think I could go through an entire IVF cycle again. We've been through four in vitro attempts. Originally, we said we would only go through one. We'll do our frozen embryos. At that point, we will have done everything biologically possible to have a child," she said. "It's a chapter we need to close.

"If the frozen ones don't work, we would continue with adoption to have a second child," she said. "We feel very strongly about that."

The microwave chirped. The baby in her arms gurgled and waved his tiny fists. His bottle was ready.

"He's so cute. He looks just like Bill," she said. "Of course, I'm not partial, am I?"

They all kept one eye on the calendar. The spring of 1990 was easing into summer. The first child conceived through Jacques Cohen's embryo hatching procedure was due within weeks.

Thirty-eight weeks after her pregnancy began, Pam Roberts delivered healthy twins by caesarean section. A seven-pound, fourteen-ounce girl, named Lauren, and a seven-pound, eight-ounce boy, Ryan. They arrived at the hospital at dawn. Her obstetrician had set the date and time—April 3, 7 A.M.—weeks before. Her husband, who always hated needles, sickrooms, and the sight of his own blood, couldn't take his eyes away. "The concept of cutting open Pam and pulling out two babies was mind-boggling, irrespective of how they got there. You can look down into the incision and see the babies before they pulled them out. By that time, I had forgotten how they were conceived." Later, they learned that Cohen had not operated on their embryos. Their offspring had been part of the control group.

On his desk, Larry Roberts now kept two framed photos of his twins: one taken at conception, when they were no more than a cluster of cells; the second as newborns. There was little about conception, pregnancy, or delivery that Pam Roberts recalled with any joy. She spent the last nine weeks before the twins were born trying to run her hospital department from home, flat on her back in bed hooked up to a computerized contraction monitor at a cost of $100 a day. Her obstetrical bills for the pregnancy and delivery totaled about $14,000. "It was like one hurdle, then another hurdle, then another. Now we look at the babies and think they are growing so fast. It was all worth it, especially now, because the babies are becoming two little people. They have impacted our lives in such a neat way. I see so many things in my husband that I never knew he was capable of doing or being or feeling."

She would resign from the hospital and become a part-time consultant.

"I think about Jacques Cohen a lot," she said. "I think about quiet Jacques, in the background, who is really the purveyor of these miracles. I wonder if Jacques has any idea of what a neat thing he has done. I thought about him this morning because Lauren was laughing and talking. She is starting to wave. There is an incredible moment when your children start to look at you and they realize who you are and smile."

On May 3, after 12 hours of labor, Lisa Boone delivered a healthy daughter, Lucy-Marie, by caesarean section. She had been prepared for weeks. "I had lists of everything I was going to take into labor in my little labor bag, and lists of things that were going with me to my hospital room. Those were two separate bags. I had them all packed a week before I was due. I had the baby's room all ready, I guess about five weeks before she was born." Her husband the malpractice attorney never left her side. "He charted my contractions and my baby's heartbeat," she said fondly. From the clinic, the Boones learned that their daughter had started life as one of Cohen's experimental "hatched" embryos. "A lot of women have dreams about having an unhealthy baby. I never did," she said. "It was almost as though I took for granted that this was an immaculate conception and I was assured of having a healthy, wonderful baby. I am a very anxious person. I worry about everything, but I didn't worry about that." Lisa Boone would resign from her full-time job so that she could spend more time with Lucy-Marie. Already they were making plans to expand their family with the two frozen embryos left in storage at the clinic. They hoped to revive them in the new year.

So far, only one other healthy baby had developed to term from an embryo that Cohen had surgically altered under the microscope—a baby boy born only days before the Booneses' baby girl. The infants' safe delivery, the culmination of the clinical trial, ended months of quiet anxiety.

Massey and Kort expected the first to be a normal birth and a healthy child, but, unlike their practice in the past, there would be no televised press conference to announce the successful birth and their medical feat. They instructed their public relations firm to withhold the public announcements. There would be no press releases, no reports in the medical journals, no news stories in *The Atlanta Constitution* or *The New York Times*. For the time being, they would keep it among the medical community. This trial had sobered the medicine men.

12

Take-Home Baby

David Parr held on to both sides of the doorway and leaned as far into the embryo laboratory as he dared without actually crossing the threshold and contaminating the sterile area. Somewhere inside were the four embryos that he and his wife had created almost a year ago.

The embryos had been frozen on October 4, 1989. Now it was July 26, 1990. Susan Parr waited for them under a blue quilt on the transfer table. When they arrived that morning, Susan or David had not yet been told how many embryos had survived the 10 months submerged in liquid nitrogen. It had taken the Parrs that long to work up the nerve for another attempt at laboratory conception. The acrimony of infertility had pushed them to the brink of divorce. That the Parrs had returned at all for their embryos was a testament to the couple's endurance.

"I have been going constantly for three years—fertility drugs, laparoscopies, in vitro. My body wore down. A lot of it is the drugs but a lot of it is you: your self-image, your weight, the stress. I was one of those pleasing kinds of people. Now I could give a damn about anyone else. This is something we are doing for ourselves," Susan said. The thirty-three-year-old auditor had brown eyes and thick brown hair with red highlights. She had met her husband in a college philosophy class and married after graduation, and had been married a dozen years. She spent her working life monitoring how public officials managed government money. She brought that same sense of proper procedure to her pursuit of pregnancy.

David, thirty-four, was a sales rep who had moved so many times that he liked to say he was from nowhere. He was short and almost bald. A fringe of brown hair crowned his head like a monk's tonsure. He was easy to overlook, easy to underestimate. He ran his own business and he snapped his fingers when he talked.

"I don't give up until the last act," he said. "She anticipates failure. She doesn't seem to understand that a crucial part of the deal is to maintain a good attitude until somebody smacks you in the face. Her emotional needs are enormous. Like I need to be more present, more agreeable, more there. Support. Support. I don't know how much is a crutch and how much is real. She gets flowers and a little gift whether the pregnancy test is positive or negative."

Their medical file was as thick as *Webster's New Collegiate Dictionary*. Infertility had never been something they worried about. She had gotten pregnant in college and had an abortion. She had her first infertility test in the spring of 1987. The doctor diagnosed severe endometriosis. She also had a hormonal defect. Given the chance, her body now killed his sperm. By summer, she was on fertility drugs. By early winter, she had undergone her first laparoscopy. By the following spring, they tried artificial insemination for the first of seven times.

Her insurance coverage, which would cover three attempts at IVF, went into effect on January 1, 1989. Four days later, she had her first appointment with Carlene Elsner at RBA. In March, the Parrs started the first of several attempts at in vitro fertilization. Jacques Cohen and Graham Wright made 13 embryos for them. Cohen surgically "hatched" them to no effect; they survived the procedure, but did not implant. Wright froze the surplus. Until now, they had been sitting in Dewar No. 2 under the lab bench at Reproductive Biology Associates. The parking space cost a total of $420.

"Nobody pipedreamed us," David said. "There weren't any

rose-colored glasses. I am amazed at what they can do. I am amazed at what they can't do. They can enhance your sperm and take your eggs and make embryos. They can freeze them and thaw them and operate on them. But when they put them back, it is like they throw them at the wall. If they stick, it's spaghetti."

After so many failures, he had contacted several adoption attorneys and attended an adoption conference.

"If you want a baby, you buy a baby. That's all there is to it. They say twenty-five thousand dollars is the going price for a healthy, white baby. Most people don't want to shell out the bucks for a baby. It's crude. But what are we doing here?"

The day before the embryo transfer, Susan got a call from the clinic's finance manager. The clinic routinely required payment in advance, and their check had bounced. David had sold stock to cover the expense, but the bank was in no hurry to transfer the funds from one account to another. As tactfully as possible, the finance manager made it clear that if that check didn't clear in time, neither would the embryos.

Michael Tucker had pulled their embryos from the storage tank the night before. The lab was deserted. Evening rush hour had already stalled traffic on the nearby superhighway. He ran the water in the sink. While it warmed, he inseminated a set of eggs left over from a couple who had undergone a GIFT procedure at lunch hour. When the water reached precisely 31 degrees Centigrade, he filled a metal carafe.

Tucker rolled Dewar No. 2 clear of the bench, opened the lid, and, as the mist roiled across the floor, rattled through the long, narrow canisters inside with a pair of tongs, looking for canister No. 9 and canister No. 3. Each canister was only slightly larger than a riverboat cigar. He found the first ampule, checked the name against his records, and plunged it into the water bath. He looked the other way. "I've had these explode on me," he said. He customarily thawed first the embryo least likely to survive. That way he could save a couple's best chance for last. "This is always the nervy bit. Will it or won't it be there? Will it or won't it survive?" He siphoned the fluid from the ampule onto the microscope stage. "Ah, there it is. It doesn't look too bad. It's intact."

Three of the embryo's four cells appeared healthy enough to survive. He retrieved a second ampule, thawed it, and in a few minutes found another healthy embryo. All four of its cells appeared undamaged.

"I am going to make the executive decision not to thaw any more," Tucker said. Those embryos Tucker left in storage would be saved in case the Parrs needed to try again later. "Tomorrow, when I have two dead embryos and none to transfer, I'll regret this. Leaving them overnight is a bit of an acid test."

By 8:30 A.M. the next day, the two embryos appeared to have resumed their retarded development. The two-cell had become three. The four-cell had become five. However, they were recovering from the shock of the thaw unusually slowly. Tucker had four cases to handle that morning. He counted on his fingers: one endometriosis, one male factor, one blocked tube, then the Parrs. Graham Wright and Sharon Wiker were handling egg collections.

While he waited for the Parrs, Tucker inspected the two eggs he had inseminated for another couple the day before. There was no fertilization. The couple to whom the eggs belonged had signed a consent form allowing him to perform partial zona dissection on any eggs that did not fertilize, but Tucker decided on a different procedure.

He would try to inject a single sperm into the egg. The couple had not given their consent for this experiment, nor had they had been asked. The experiment had not been reviewed by an institutional review board, as was usually customary. Tucker had been practicing on old eggs. Three times he had fertilized eggs which then appeared to divide like a normal embryo. But he had never tried to transfer any of them to a patient. If what he tried this morning produced an embryo, Tucker said he would freeze it for an otherwise routine transfer at a later date, as if they were no different from any other embryo.

"I suppose it is a bit naughty doing it this way. But if, after several months, I've gotten absolutely nowhere, I will have saved a lot of time filling out protocols and forms," he said.

The microtools, which seemed so easy to make when Henry Malter was operating the forge, kept breaking. Tucker could not get the injection needle—finer than a human hair—to shear properly. Three times he tried and failed. He tapped his fingers on the counter.

"This is a little bit frustrating," he said.

After 20 minutes, he inserted his best effort into one arm of the micromanipulator and put a holding pipette into the other. He pooled some of the husband's sperm, left over from the day before, under the microscope. He added the two eggs.

Through the microscope, the first egg looked like an elongated vitamin capsule, sadly out of shape. The sperm cells around it hopped like water fleas. Tucker siphoned several sperm cells into the beveled hollow of the injection needle and tried to pierce the lower end of the egg. The needle kept sliding off the tough membrane. He tried and failed several times, then moved the needle to the top of the egg and tried again. "The needle is not sharp enough to pierce the zona," Tucker said. Another 20 minutes had passed.

He inserted a new needle. Its tip was too narrow to take up the entire sperm cell. He improvised. He made the hole first, then withdrew the needle. He snapped off its tip, scooped up two sperm, and inserted them through the original slit in the zona. They were left wriggling inside.

He repeated the procedure with the second egg; he made a hole with the needle, withdrew it, then snapped off the tip. He picked up three sperm and, using the same hole, tried to place them inside the egg. As he tried to expel them from the needle, he inadvertently exerted too much pressure. The egg instantly expanded to twice its size like a balloon ready to explode. Tucker quickly released the pressure and the egg shrank to its normal size. The bubble did not burst, and it seemed to have suffered no visible damage.

He was embarrassed by the possibility that he had damaged the egg during the experiment. "In this case, the woman has already had some sperm and eggs put back inside her. That is her best chance of getting pregnant. So in a way these eggs are not so crucial, really," he said. He slid them back into the incubator. The Parrs had arrived. He took out another dish containing their thawed embryos and readied them for the transfer.

"All right, rock and roll," said Susan as the two embryos appeared on the monitor screen. One looked like a four-leaf clover. Tucker carefully explained the state of the two embryos to them. Both embryos appeared healthy and, recovered from the shock of the thaw, had started to divide normally.

"It is cleaving? Actually cleaving?" Susan asked. Tucker nodded. "What are my odds with two being put back?"

Tucker shook his head. "I'm not a betting man, really. I give you a twenty or a twenty-five percent chance."

"If you don't roll the dice, you can't get the double sixes," she said. David walked over and kissed her.

Carlene Elsner slipped into the room, donned her sterile gloves, and turned on her headlamp. She looked at the screen. "Even one of those will make a baby," she said. The transfer took only a few seconds. Tucker took the catheter back into the laboratory and checked it under the microscope.

"Okay," he called back.

David stepped into the spotlight cast by the light on Elsner's brow and tap-danced. "You can do your dance after she's a pregnant lady," Carlene Elsner said.

Susan Parr parked her black Alfa Romeo at the end of the driveway, threw the keys into her purse, and strode into the house through the garage past her husband's basement sales office. She was near tears. For two weeks the two embryos had incubated inside her. At 10:30 A.M., she had her blood drawn for a pregnancy test. The clinic was to have called at 3 P.M. with the results. She fled the house before the phone could ring. From her back pain and muscle cramps, she was certain she was not pregnant. She couldn't face it again. She couldn't bear to hear the bad news over the telephone.

She idled an hour among the lipsticks and blush brushes at Rich's department store. There, experimenting with beauty masks, she could keep back the tears. "I can't hear that voice again saying 'Susan, it's negative.' I've lost track of the number of negative tests I've had. I feel so cheated and frustrated. I want to lie down and bury myself. I am at the end," she said. "It will be negative, I know."

David stolidly watched her come through the door, his arms folded across his chest. She crossed the distance between them.

"I hugged him and told him I was sorry it didn't work out. We were a team this time and we could be proud of that. We tried and that was what counted. Maybe next time it would work," she said. They had been through this so many times that they both knew all the words by heart.

He left a magazine for her in the kitchen. "Go look at your magazine," he said.

On the table, he had placed the August issue of *Life* magazine. Splashed across its cover was a color photograph of a seven-week-old embryo, its tiny fingers splayed across its chest. The caption read: HOW LIFE BEGINS. THE FIRST PICTURES EVER. David had taped a note on the cover: IN YOU! I LOVE U. Next to the magazine there were a dozen roses in a vase, couched in baby's breath.

"She stared at me and I stared at her. She didn't get it. I said, 'You are pregnant.' I had tears welling up in my eyes. She thought I was lying."

When it dawned on her, she fell to her knees and wept.

"We can make life," David said. "Now we have to make it well enough so it can nurture itself. It's a kind of unnatural act of God. We had these frozen embryos. They come back from death, from the frost. Now we are looking down the barrel of normalcy. What we have done is go through all this hell to get back to normal—if you call raising a family normal these days. We're still leery. It can be like a wisp of wind that brushes your ear and then is gone."

A month later, Susan and David Parr had their first ultrasound scan of the developing fetus. They did not know yet whether one or both of the embryos had implanted. Her hormone levels were high, and she had been warned to expect twins. She would find out how many hearts there were within her.

Already she felt herself transformed. She felt comforted and, at last, consoled. "The feeling you have is not desperation," she said. "The feeling of wanting to be pregnant—to want a child—has been so strong for so long. *Yearning* is the word. I tell myself now that my heart is not going to break in two. I have to catch myself and remind myself I am pregnant. I was always a loner, always independent. The isolation of infertility has made me even more of a loner. It has changed me. It has changed us. Our relationship. Our social life.

"I keep wondering what it will be like to hold my own baby," she said. "The fetal heartbeat will do a lot to make it real for me. One day soon, I will come home at the end of the day and my child will be there. And I will feel so rich."

She hoped for twins. She had signed up for Cohen's experiment with that in mind so many months before.

"I'll take what I can get. If I get twins, I'll be ecstatic. If I don't get twins, I'll be overjoyed. All I want is a healthy baby. I don't know what my numbers are supposed to be. I don't know the rules to this one. I don't have a standard to judge my performance. It's frightening and exciting."

When they arrived at the clinic, they were ushered into a smaller waiting room, away from the contingent of infertile couples at the main lobby. A young couple emerged from the ultrasound room arm in arm. The newly expectant mother waved a damp Polaroid photograph in her free hand and beamed. "We got a heartbeat," she said. She proffered the photograph. The fetus inside her—six weeks and six days old—was less than nine millimeters long. "Well, it is a little blob," she said. "It is our little blob."

From the doorway, the ultrasonographer beckoned to the Parrs. "How many did you have transferred? Two?"

She made some notations in the file. Susan climbed onto the table, and David found a corner out of the way. The technician inserted the ultrasound probe. A black-and-silver shimmer appeared on the screen. At its center, no more distinct than a wisp of cumulus cloud, a white sliver pulsed rhythmically, framed in the crosshairs.

"You can see the little flutter of the heartbeat," the technician said. "Look at the screen. You made it. Don't cry, you'll make me cry." Susan leaned up and stared at the screen. Her face reddened with tears. "We are seeing a singleton with a heartbeat," the technician said. Susan was about seven weeks pregnant, but the embryo was actually almost old enough to celebrate its first birthday.

"We are doing a singleton?" Susan asked.

"A singleton, yes."

"That little flutter? That's a heartbeat?" Susan asked. She looked across at David.

The technician let them absorb the view. "It's about twice as fast as your heartbeat, Susan. You did it." She gave them a photograph.

The technician directed them down an unfamiliar hallway to a small examination room where Carlene Elsner would meet with them. "We've never been down here before. I guess this is where we graduate," Susan said.

David stared at the photograph. "We've got a little thumper," he said.

Elsner only took a few minutes to examine Susan, then reminded them both that they still had two embryos in storage. They couldn't stay there forever. "We would prefer that you use them and not your daughter," Elsner said. She got up to leave.

Susan tried to stay calm. "What do I do now? What are the rules?"

"The rules of the game are that it is time for you to call an obstetrician," Elsner replied. "Who's going to deliver the baby?"

"I have no idea." Susan looked lost. After becoming so expert in the technology of conception, the Parrs were neophytes at the business of pregnancy. Her voice tightened. "I've never gotten this far before. I don't know the rules. Am I high risk? Do I need a special obstetrician? Do I need somebody who has had experience with in vitro babies? What should I do?"

Elsner leaned against the wall and looked amused. "You should start thinking about nursery colors and cribs. You don't need me anymore. You are a boring, normal pregnant lady now."

By the fall of 1990, 28 women had safely delivered babies who started life as one of Jacques Cohen's experimental "hatched" embryos. There were an additional 40 fetuses at different stages of development in 29 other expectant mothers who had volunteered for his clinical trial. One set of identical twins had miscarried. Tests revealed that they had grown from the same embryo. Perhaps they had been caught, as Cohen had worried months before, half in and half out of the hole he had opened in the embryo's protective membrane. In that constriction, a single fetus became two.

It was difficult to know what precisely the embryologist had learned. Clinically speaking, he had only discovered enough about the effects of embryo micromanipulation by the end of his experiment to know that he had to find out more. "It doesn't seem to work for anyone else," Cohen said. In Atlanta, Michael Tucker's clinical trial had only just begun. In New York, Cohen began another controlled trial of the embryo "hatching" procedure. This time, Cohen waited until each embryo was older and sturdier before making a hole in its membrane. And he would make a larger hole. The first four women who volunteered for the procedure became pregnant.

For the time being, all Cohen could say was that he had done no harm. What so far had failed to bring about the consistent results he hoped for, however, had succeeded in other ways. From his hatching, slurping, and schlepping, others learned they could safely cut and pierce the human embryo without affecting its ability to become a healthy child. With that assurance, others turned his techniques to their own ends. What Cohen and his volunteers had contributed was their willingness to gamble with the lives they made, to assume a risk that by reason of prudence, politics, or law others avoided. The embryologists inched toward understanding. From fleeting hints and educated guesswork, they felt their way around the mystery that was creation.

Jacques Cohen, who took such care with the thousands of embryos conceived in his laboratories, rarely saw the children who grew from the microscopic clusters of cells he created. Cohen and his assistants anxiously charted the health of each new developing fetus, studying its ultrasound scans and amniocentesis results carefully, with the knowledge that any defect would trigger a flurry of postmortem exams and laboratory tests. As soon as he was confident each fetus was healthy, however, Cohen seemed to lose interest, often at the very moment the parents themselves realized that they had created more than an act of faith. They were all accomplices: Cohen had created viable human embryos; the parents made of them healthy babies, and the babies would make a life.

"My aim is to make the women pregnant," Cohen said. "You think Cohen who makes babies is not interested in them? I am very touched by some of them, but across the board I see them as numbers.

"Maybe deep down, I'm not interested in babies," Cohen said. He laughed. "I see a lot of babies. They come and show me their babies. I am delighted to see them, but I have observed that the nurses and the doctors are more delighted than I am. I am more distanced. I don't want children myself. It would jeopardize too much of my life. Maybe in ten years."

He drew a long breath. He was caught by the memory of the couples he glimpsed every day across the threshold of his embryo laboratory—men and women crippled not by a physical disability, but by the acid of doubt, anger, and shame.

"For me, it is not so much the baby," he said. "I want to stop the agony of the patient. I am much more delighted that these patients are no longer suffering. When I go to these clinic reunions—these IVF birthday parties—the pleasure for me is to see that the couples have lost this kind of insanity. It was more than that they wanted a baby so badly. There was this imperfection they felt—the thought that they are themselves imperfect. They have lost that. I am overjoyed.

"In a couple of years, people will think everything I am doing here is horribly ridiculous. That's the way science is. You know, a real scientist—a real basic research embryologist who works only with laboratory animals—looks down on me. But I have seen things they have never seen in the human."

Appendix

Selected Bibliography

Andrews, Lori. *Between Strangers: Surrogate Mothers, Expectant Fathers and Brave New Babies*. Harper & Row (1989).

Australian In Vitro Fertilization Collaborative Group. "High Incidence of Pre-term Births and Early Losses in Pregnancy After In Vitro Fertilization." *British Medical Journal*, vol. 291 (1985): 1160–1163.

Baruch, Elaine Hoffman, Amadeo F. D'Adamo, Jr., and Joni Seagar, editors. *Embryos, Ethics and Women's Rights*. Harrington Park Press (1988).

Bishop, Jerry E. and Michael Waldholz. *Genome*. Simon & Schuster (1990).

Brown, Lesley and John. *Our Miracle Called Louise: A Parents' Story*. Paddington Press (1979).

Charlesworth, Max. "Life, Death, Genes, and Ethics: 1989 Boyer Lectures." Australian Broadcasting Corporation (1989).

Cohen, Jacques, Gary W. DeVane, Carlene W. Elsner, Carole B. Fehilly, Hilton I. Kort, Joe B. Massey, Thomas G. Turner, Jr. "Cryopreservation of zygotes and early cleaved human embryos." *Fertility and Sterility*, vol. 45, no. 5 (1988) : 283–287.

Cohen, Jacques, Alexis Adler, Mina Alikani, Henry Malter, Beth Talansky. "Enhancement of Fertilization and Implantation by Micromanipulation." *The Proceedings of the First International Meeting on Preimplantation Genetics*. Plenum Press (1991).

Cohen, Jacques, R. F. Simons, Carole Fehilly, and Robert Edwards.

"Factors Affecting Survival and Implantation of Cryopreserved Human Embryos." *Journal of In Vitro Fertilization and Embryo Transfer*. 3:53 (1986).

Cohen, Jacques, Carlene Elsner, Hilton Kort, Henry E. Malter, Joe Massey, Mary Pat Mayer, and Klaus E. Weimer. "Impairment of the Hatching Process Following In Vitro Fertilization in the Human and Improvement of Implantation by Assisting Hatching Using Micromanipulation." *Human Reproduction*, vol. 5, no. 1 (1990) : 7–13.

Cohen, Jacques, Robert Edwards, Carole Fehilly, Simon Fishel, Jonathan Hewitt, Jean Purdy, George Rowland, Patrick Steptoe, and John Webster. "In Vitro Fertilization: A Treatment for Male Infertility." *Fertility and Sterility*, vol. 43, no. 3 (1985) : 422–432.

Corea, Gena. *The Mother Machine*. The Women's Press Ltd. (1988).

Dunstan, G. R., and Mary J. Seller. *The Status of the Human Embryo: Perspectives from a Moral Tradition*. King Edward's Hospital Fund for London, Oxford University Press (1988).

Dyson, Anthony, and John Harris, editors. *Experiments on Embryos: Social Ethics and Public Policy*. Routledge (1990).

Edwards, Robert. *Life Before Birth: Reflections on the Embryo Debate*. Century Hutchinson Ltd. (1989).

Elias, Sherman, and George J. Annas. *Reproductive Genetics and The Law*. Year Book Medical Publishers Inc. (1987).

Ethics Committee of The American Fertility Society. "Ethical Considerations of the New Reproductive Technologies. *Fertility and Sterility*, vol. 53, no. 6, Supplement 2 (1990).

Ford, Norman M. *When Did I Begin? Conception of the Human Individual in History, Philosophy and Science*. Cambridge University Press (1988).

Gordon, Jon W., Larry Grunfield, G. John Garrisi, Daniel Navot, and Neri Laufer. "Successful microsurgical removal of a pronucleus from tripronuclear human zygotes." *Fertility and Sterility*, vol. 52, no. 3 (1989) : 367–372.

Grobstein, Clifford. *Science and the Unborn*. Basic Books Inc. (1988).

Gunning, Jennifer. "Human IVF, Embryo Research, Fetal Tissue for Research and Treatment and Abortion: International Information." Department of Health, London: Her Majesty's Stationery Office (1990).

Handyside, Alan, E. H. Kontogianni, K. Hardy, and R. M. L. Winston. "Pregnancies from Biopsied Human Preimplantation Embryos Sexed by Y-specific DNA Amplification." *Nature*, vol. 344 (1990) : 768–770.

Jones, Jr., Howard W., Georgeanna Seegar Jones, Gary D. Hodgen, and Sev Rosenwaks. "In Vitro Fertilization: Norfolk." Waverly Press (1986).

Lancaster, Paul A. L. "Congenital Malformations After In Vitro Fertilization." *The Lancet* (December 12, 1987).

Malter, Henry E., and Jacques Cohen. "Embryonic Development After Microsurgical Repair of Polyspermic Human Zygotes." *Fertility and Sterility*, vol. 52, no. 3 (1989) : 373–380.

Malter, Henry E., Beth Talansky, Jon Gordon, and Jacques Cohen. "Monospermy and Polyspermy After Partial Zona Dissection of Reinseminated Human Oocytes." *Gamete Research*, vol. 23, no. 4 (1989) : 377–386.

Malter, Henry E., Jacques Cohen. "Partial Zona Dissection of the Human Oocyte: A Method Using Nontraumatic Micromanipulation to Assist Zona Pellucida Penetration." *Fertility and Sterility*, vol. 51, no. 1 (1989) : 139–148.

Ng, Soon-Chye, Ariff Bongso, Sheau-Ine Chang, Henry Sathanantham, and Shan Ratnam. "Transfer of Human Sperm into the Perivitelline Space of Human Oocytes After Zona Drilling or Zona Puncture." *Fertility and Sterility*, vol. 52, no. 1 (1989) : 73–78.

Ratcliff, Kathryn Strother, et al., editors. *Healing Technology: Feminist Perspectives*. The University of Michigan Press (1989).

Robertson, John A. "In the Beginning: The Legal Status of Early Human Embryos." *Virginia Law Review*, vol. 76, no. 3 (1990) : 437–517.

Rothman, Barbara Katz. *Recreating Motherhood: Ideology and Technology in a Patriarchal Society*. W. W. Norton & Co. (1989).

Saunders, Douglas M., and Paul Lancaster. "The Wider Perinatal Significance of the Australian In Vitro Fertilization Data Collection Program." *American Journal of Perinatology*, vol. 6, no. 2 (1989) : 252–257.

Spallone, Patricia. *Beyond Conception: The New Politics of Reproduction*. Bergin & Harvey Publishers Inc. (1989).

The Randolph W. Thrower Symposium: Genetics and the Law. *Emory Law Journal*, vol. 39, no. 3 (1990).

Trounson, Alan. "Current Perspectives of In Vitro Fertilization and Embryo Transfer." *Clinical Reproduction and Fertility*, vol. 1 (1982).

United Kingdom, Department of Health and Social Security. "Report of the Committee of Inquiry into Human Fertilization and Embryology." Warnock Committee (1984).

U.S. Congress, Office of Technology Assessment. "Artificial Insem-